D0502548

WEIGHT LOSS
SUCCESS
WITHOUT DIETING

Thank You! Dear George,

*My husband and I have been following the Healthiest Way of Eating plan with **The World's Healthiest Foods** for three weeks now. In that time, we have basically experienced a miracle.*

I have lost 5 lbs. and he has lost 6 lbs. since beginning the plan. The best part of doing your plan is that we aren't hungry. In the past, we have been able to stick to a diet for about 2 weeks before we gave up, usually with a binge. But on the plan, neither of us feel as if we are starving. We are generally not missing the foods we used to eat.

Your recipes are absolutely delicious and satisfying. We both feel that the Healthiest Way of Eating is something we can do for the rest of our lives. Thank you for creating this plan. It has made a huge difference in our lives.

Sincerely,
Sylvia

WEIGHT LOSS SUCCESS

WITHOUT DIETING

True Stories About Losing Weight
with the World's Healthiest Foods

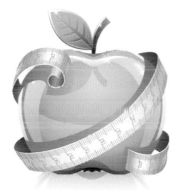

George Mateljan

Author of *The World's Healthiest Foods:*
Essential Guide for the Healthiest Way of Eating

Books by George Mateljan

The World's Healthiest Foods:
Essential Guide for the Healthiest Way of Eating

300 Secrets:
You Should Know about the Healthiest Way of Eating

Cooking Without Fat

Baking Without Fat

Healthy Living Cuisine

Healthier Eating Guide

Natural Foods Cookbook

Healthiest Way of Cooking with George DVD

George Mateljan Foundation
PO Box 25801
Seattle, WA 09125-1301

Back Book Cover Photos:

Poached Halibut with Fennel and Cauliflower – page 152
Citrus Spinach Salad With Shrimp – page 132
10-Minute Fresh Berry Dessert with Yogurt and Chocolate – page 180

Weight Loss Success – Without Dieting
1st Edition
ISBN 978-0-9769185-3-0
Printed in Canada

From George Mateljan

Have you been trying to lose weight but been unsuccessful? If so, I believe I have the answer for you. I think you have been eating the wrong foods.

Have you had those extra pounds seemingly creep up on you with no apparently obvious reason? It's not as if you feel like you've been eating more than usual, and certainly not enough to show up so strikingly on the scale.

Most all of us have experienced this at least once in our lifetime. It takes us by surprise and leaves us in a slight state of shock because it doesn't seem as though we have done anything to deserve this extra poundage.

I am no exception. Like millions of others, I have personally experienced the rollercoaster ride of losing and regaining a large amount of weight (over 50 pounds). Because it is such a widespread problem, there doesn't seem to be any area of health in which there is more time, effort, and money spent than in the area of weight loss. So even though those of us who are trying to lose weight decrease food intake and exercise more, long-term weight loss still seems to elude many of us. The common scenario is to initially lose weight but soon gain it back. In fact, in about 95% of cases people regain all the weight they lost, and oftentimes end up heavier than when they started!

Preventing this weight loss roller coaster and helping you to find a way to enjoy the right foods that can help you get and stay slim and healthy is what this book is all about. Very few people can sustain a starvation-type diet or diets that are nutritionally imbalanced and deprive the body of the important nutrients it needs to function optimally.

Scientific studies continue to demonstrate that among all lifestyle factors, no single factor is more important to our health than the food we eat. The concept of practicing a healthier way of eating can easily be overlooked as a means to resolving our problem of being overweight. Yet, focusing on the intake of foods that are nutrient-rich foods, low in calories, and very satisfying—like the *World's Healthiest Foods*—can prove to be one of the most powerful ways to affect better health and *Weight Loss Success.*

Enjoying more whole foods like the *World's Healthiest Foods* can be our key to change. As we become increasingly conscious of calories, salt, sugar, and fat that is contained in pre-packaged, processed, refined, nutrient-poor foods, and fast foods we can start looking at them in a different way. We will then be less drawn in by their image of convenience, fun, and stimulation, rather seeing them for what they really are—foods that potentially harmful (they don't nourish us with all the nutrients we need) and are associated with epidemic proportions of obesity as well as reduced immune function, increased risk of heart disease as well as elevated blood sugar levels, which increases our proclivity for diabetes. Enjoying the World's Healthiest Foods is a great way to overcome your desire for nutrient-poor foods.

When I lost my weight, I gave most of the credit to eating more of the *World's Healthiest Vegetables* because even among the *World's Healthiest Foods*, they are the foods that are the most nutrient-rich and lowest in calories. Extra helpings of these foods helped control my hunger and prevented me from indulging in excess calories, which caused me to gain weight. In addition to losing weight and keeping it off, eating this way ultimately helped me improve my health. In this book I share with you the *World's Healthiest Vegetables* and my secrets of how I prepare them to be so enjoyable that it is easy to make them the centerpiece of my meals. When I did this I lost over 50 pounds without dieting, and I have kept it off for over ten years. Many of our Readers have had similar experiences, and so can you!

George Mateljan

Contents

What are the World's Healthiest Foods

The leading prestigious British medical journal, Lancet, reports that 50% of the U.S. population will be obese by 2030 unless we start eating the right foods. It was George's desire to find the "right foods"—health-promoting foods—that inspired him to travel to over 80 countries and experience the cuisines of different cultures renowned for their health and longevity. This led to his creating his list of the World's Healthiest Foods and writing the best-selling book, The World's Healthiest Foods: Essential Guide for the Healthiest Way of Eating. These are foods exceptionally rich in vitamins, minerals, protein, fiber, phytonutrients (see page 48) in relation to the amount of calories they contain. Readers reported that eating more of the World's Healthiest Foods not only helped them to improve their health but lose weight as well!

Why We Have an Apple on the Cover

Apples have traditionally been the symbol of good health. Increasing scientific evidence of apples' health-promoting properties continues to support the old adage "an apple a day keeps the doctor away." According to a study by Cornell University, one medium apple may contain only about 6 mg of vitamin C, however it has enough other antioxidants to produce as much antioxidant activity as 1,500 mg of vitamin C. Another study found that a daily consumption of apples significantly helped subjects experience weight loss success. One medium apple is rich in fiber and contains only 81 calories for a perfect snack or treat anytime of day.

How to Benefit Most from This Book

The book shares with you how an approach to eating that emphasizes nutrient-rich foods, such as the *World's Healthiest Foods*, can help you on your journey to *Weight Loss Success*, without dieting and deprivation.

In Section 1, I'll reveal that the key feature of foods that help promote weight loss and health is nutrient-richness. I explain what this term means, provide you with examples of nutrient-rich foods, and discuss the benefits of the key nutrients in which the *World's Healthiest Foods* are concentrated.

In Section 2, you'll find the *Calorie-Lowering Plan*, menus that you can use for 4 weeks that take the guesswork out of designing meals for health and healthy weight. Included here you'll find all the recipes that you'll prepare for these 4 weeks plus practical tips that can help you in your continued healthy weight loss.

In Section 3, I describe important ways that nutrient-rich foods support weight loss success. Here you can discover how they can help you manage adverse food reactions, promote energy production and optimal metabolism, support digestive and liver health, maintain balanced blood sugar levels, and curb inflammation.

I've also compiled a section of Q&As that address various topics associated with *Weight Loss Success*. These include the role of calorie intake in weight management, the difference between nutrient-rich and energy-rich foods, and so much more. You can find these in Section 4.

INTRODUCTION

The recommendations in this book are designed to help you replicate the experiences of Readers like Astrida who lost 32 pounds and wrote to us saying: "The *World's Healthiest Foods* are the possible cure for the American problem of obesity." Other Readers have noted that they experienced weight loss as great as 30, 40, 50, and even 100 pounds or more through dietary changes that involved consumption of more of the *World's Healthiest Foods*.

This is not a diet book. Rather, it's a book on how to discover foods that are both nutrient-rich and low in calories to help you improve your health and increase your chances of losing weight—a necessary combination for the weight loss success stories that were reported to us by our Readers.

In Chapter 1 you can read e-mails from over 30 of our many Readers who ate more of the *World's Healthiest Foods* and lost weight without dieting. They found that this was an effective way to lose weight and gain greater energy and better health at the same time.

Why the World's Healthiest Foods May Help You Improve Health and Lose Weight

The *World's Healthiest Foods* are nutrient-rich, which means they contain the greatest number of nutrients for the least number of calories. They are packed with vitamins, minerals, protein, fiber, and phytonutrients. Because the *World's Healthiest Foods* are such health-promoting foods, some Readers found that their blood pressure, cholesterol, and sugar levels were reduced and that they experienced better sleep and memory. And they also lost weight. In other words they became healthier and lost weight at the same time—a winning combination.

Losing Weight Without Dieting

We were surprised (as our Readers may have been as well) that the goal of improved health also resulted in weight loss — and for some it was quite dramatic weight loss! That's why we call this *"Weight Loss Success—Without Dieting"* as they lost weight without focusing on losing weight. And what could be a better way to lose weight.

We believe one of the keys to success is the emphasis of our Healthiest Way of Eating on enjoying the W*orld's Healthiest* Vegetables (see page 55). That's because the *World's Healthiest Vegetables* are incredibly nutrient-rich, with many being extremely low in calories. They seem to be at the core of healthy weight loss.

Therefore my goal in this book is to share more about the lowest calorie, nutrient-rich *World's Healthiest Vegetables* and easy ways to prepare them so they taste great. This way if they taste great you'll want to eat more. And as you do, you'll be supporting your overall well-being.

How to Minimize Your Calories

To lose weight you need to minimize your caloric intake and consume fewer calories than you burn. To optimize your health you need to maximize your nutritional intake. I believe this is the one-two punch to achieve a healthy body and healthy weight loss. The *World's Healthiest Vegetables* are among the best foods to fill this bill. They are the *World's Healthiest Foods* that have the greatest number of nutrients for the least number of calories. In fact most of them are so low in calories you can eat as much of them as you like, that is if you enjoy them without the addition of fatty dressings or oils. And they are also rich in fiber—one important component to helping you feel satiated and satisfied after a meal. Combine them with the other *World's Healthiest Foods* as a support team (such as in our *Calorie Lowering Plan*), to help meet your daily nutritional requirements.

As our Readers discovered, a healthy body and healthy weight loss are actually not two separate goals. If you don't nourish your body with the nutrients you need (vitamins, minerals, protein, fiber, omega-3 fatty acids, phytonutrients, and others), your body won't function optimally. And if you feel tired, fatigued, stressed, you will overeat because you mind is genetically programmed to eat until you get all the nutrients you need. Your body therefore tells you to keep eating because even if you are full your body is still starved for nutrients.

How I Make the World's Healthiest Vegetables Taste Great

It may not come as a surprise that the *World's Healthiest Vegetables* are among the lowest calorie foods. Although people may know that vegetables are weight-loss super stars, they often don't find them enjoyable enough to regularly include them as a large part of their meals. Perhaps one of the primary reasons that only 5% of the people who lose weight by following a diet keep that weight off is because no matter how much we want to improve our health or lose weight, we won't continue to do something that is not enjoyable.

Not only is good taste and enjoyment an important motivating factor in making a change to healthier eating, but in today's society, it is also important that preparation takes a minimal amount of time. This is the winning combination that I have developed over the years — great-tasting *World's Healthiest Vegetables* that take minimal cooking time. The new cooking methods and recipes presented here are quick and easy (most *World's Healthiest Vegetables* take only 5-7 minutes to prepare) with simple ingredients that are easy to find and have great flavor. And there's plenty of room for variation. Adding optional ingredients can transform a dish into an entirely new taste experience and also help make them suited them to your personal preferences.

Calorie Lowering Plan

Part of adopting a Healthiest Way of Eating lifestyle is changing old eating habits. And this is often difficult because we don't know where to start. That's why I created the *Calorie-Lowering Plan* that cuts 500 calories from a standard 2000 calorie a day menu. The Plan takes the guesswork out of preparing 4 weeks' worth of meals that will set you on your way to better health and meeting your healthy weight loss goals.

The powerful *Calorie-Lowering Plan* will help you embark on a healthy lifestyle change to healthier eating that's enjoyable and will not only help you attain your weight management goals, but also your desire for vibrant health and energy. I wanted to create for you the absolute best possible Plan that helps provide you with the maximum number of nutrients for the minimal number of calories. Everyday for 4 weeks, I will show you what foods to prepare using my mouth-watering, satisfying recipes and cooking methods to make food taste great. You will eat healthier and better foods than you ever thought possible. Following this Plan you will be eating the right foods—delicious fruits, crisp salads, high-energy vegetables, high-fiber legumes, lean protein foods, and more. In 4 weeks eating more of the *World's Healthiest Vegetables* will become a habit. You will be enjoying good carbohydrates and fats as well as lots of fiber to help you get healthier and work toward weight loss at the same time.

In the beginning, when you start on the Plan, you may feel deprived when you can't eat your favorite refined, nutrient-poor foods rich in sugar, salt, and fat. But after a couple of weeks of eating more nutrient-rich foods, I think you will find that any "craving" you had for refined, nutrient-poor foods will decrease, as they will begin to taste too sugary, too salty, and too fatty; you will then begin to enjoy the more delicate flavors of fresh, whole, nutrient-rich *World's Healthiest Vegetables* in the form of crisp salads, high-energy side vegetable dishes, and crunchy appetizers, all of which are combined with other foods that provide culinary pleasure and great nutritional value.

In this effective Healthiest Way of Eating approach to weight loss you will become empowered to control your weight loss through practicing new healthy eating habits (while also getting regular exercise). If you make the commitment to losing weight I believe this book will bring you what you are seeking. You will become more informed, feel more vitalized and powerful, and enjoy a greater level of well-being.

Supporting Your Healthier Eating Lifestyle

With this book and the WHFoods.org website always at your side you will have constant support on how to eat healthier and enjoy more of the *World's Healthiest Foods* as a regular part of your meals. The website focuses on different Foods of the Week that are in season and taste the best at that particular time of year. George's videos help you learn how to prepare the Food of the Week by demonstrating the preparation of some of the over 200 recipes found on the website. Learning easy tips from George of how to prepare the World's Healthiest Foods will inspire you do more of your cooking at home, which has been found not only to save time and money but to help improve health as well. And for additional support, you can sign up for the Weekly Newsletter as well as the Daily Tips and Recipes. You can also us on Facebook and Twitter. All of these are available to you free-of-charge.

Proceeds from this book will go towards research that will continue to help educate our Readers about the benefits of healthy eating and cooking with the World's Healthiest Foods with the goal of helping to make this a healthier world.

SECTION 1

The World's Healthiest Foods are the Cornerstone of Weight Loss Success

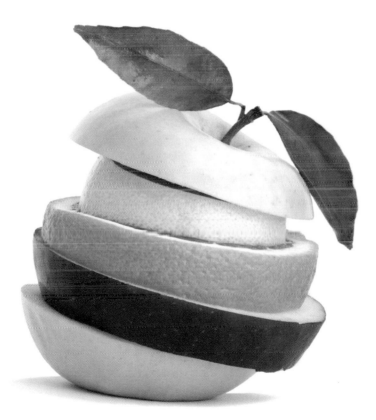

CHAPTER 1

Weight Loss Success Stories

Since I have been a small child I have been interested in healthy eating and cooking. My passion for healthy foods continued as an adult, and I have dedicated my life to helping people learn about how to eat and cook more healthfully. I have written five best-selling books about healthy foods and healthy cooking. As founder of Healthy Valley Foods I provided health-conscious people with over 300 products from recipes I created over a period of 26 years.

Over ten years ago, the George Mateljan Foundation was created with the same goal in mind. Over the years I traveled to over 80 countries, studying the eating habits of people who were renowned for their exceptional health and longevity. The result was my list of World's Healthiest Foods, the properties of which scientific studies have been showing to promote optimal health.

To help people eat and cook more healthy foods also guided the creation of our World's Healthiest Foods website (www.WHFoods.org) and *The World's Healthiest Foods: Essential Guide for the Healthiest Way of Eating* book, both of which were designed to inspire you to include more of these foods into your daily meals. I introduced my new cooking methods not only to help the foods retain more of their natural nutrients but also to make them taste great so that the path to increased energy, looking and feeling your best, and improved health could be made easier and more enjoyable. The website has helped so many people and has seen phenomenal growth over the last 10 years—it now has over 1 million unique visitors a month! It comes up #1 on a Google search for "healthiest foods" and "healthiest recipes" among many other key words and phrases, while *The World's Health-iest Foods* book has become a best seller since its publication.

During the past 10 years, I have been delighted to receive thousands of letters of gratitude from Readers who have changed their lives by enjoying a new lifestyle of eating with the World's Healthiest Foods. I am very appreciative of the time they have taken to share their stories. They have written to tell me that they have experienced greater energy, better sleep, healthier hair, clearer skin, enhanced concentration and memory, and many other signs of overall vitality. Others have also shared that eating the World's Healthiest Foods has helped their cholesterol to drop, their blood pressure to normalize, their blood sugar levels to stabilize, and their headaches to dissipate.

Not long after Readers began sharing stories about these health benefits, I also began to get letters from some Readers who reported that they believed their new way of eating with the World's Health-iest Foods also helped them to achieve a healthy weight. Because their stories inspired the writing of this book I would like to share some of them here with you. I believe their stories will be as inspirational to you as they were to me:

Readers Stories About Weight Loss

The World's Healthiest Foods is possibly the cure to the American problems of obesity. From my own experience, I decided to change my diet in the New Year. I was obese—at 5'8" I was about 240 pounds. Now six months later, I have lost 32 pounds and am still losing. I feel and look a lot better. I hope to lose another 28 pounds...and with exercise and your great recipes, I should be able to do it. THANKS A LOT! - Astrida

On May 19th of this year, my general practitioner told me my triglycerides were 374. I decided to eat my way out of poor health instead of taking drugs. As I researched the web for info on foods that would help, WHFoods.com kept popping up. Soon, I was hooked. 3 days is all it took. Ten years of chronic heartburn was gone in 3 days 40 years of allergies were gone in a week. I have lost 15 pounds and I suspect 20 pounds of body fat. Joint pain and back pain are gone. Mental clarity has increased. Memory has increased. Metabolism has increased. I am now able to run again for the first time in a decade. Acne is gone. Wounds heal in a week. Endurance has increased. Here is the amazing part, I HAVE ONLY BEEN EATING THIS WAY FOR A MONTH! – GR

One benefit I've discovered from eating high-fiber, nutrient-rich-World's Healthiest Foods is that I'm losing about 2 pounds per week without any change in my exercise habits. I don't feel deprived because I don't consider myself to be "on a diet." Thank you again for your outstanding website. Eating the right foods has changed my entire outlook on life. – Mike

The two weeks we have been on your program has proved not only to be nutritious but extremely tasty. Members of my household are for the first time eating fish and not complaining. My partner has lost half a stone in two weeks so I would just like to say a very big thank you. – Lara

Because of your great website, WHFoods, you have helped change my health for the better. I went from 24% body fat to 13% body fat. Thanks again for your generous knowledge. – GVU

Through diet and exercise I lost 170 pounds. I have your list of the World's Healthiest Foods on my refrigerator. – Mark

For more testimonials see page 240.

Readers' Stories About Weight Loss and Improved Health

While excess weight in and of itself may be cosmetically undesirable, its most serious harmful effects result from the fact that excess fat, particularly around the mid-section, greatly increases risk of developing a myriad of other health problems, including high cholesterol, high blood pressure, elevated blood sugar levels, heart disease, and stroke.

By using some of the guides, recipes, and tips from WHFoods, I've lost 40 pounds. I feel better and my thinking is more clear. I had high blood pressure but that went away when I lost the weight. – Kmuzu

Since I started eating the World's Healthiest Foods, my blood sugar has stabilized, and I have lost 50 pounds! I have truly turned my life around. – Cindy

I changed the way I ate, and I have the World's Healthiest Foods to thank. I have lost over 75 pounds. My blood pressure medication is gone. I didn't count calories and I didn't even care about portion control. – Mary

With your help, I have lost 80 pounds; my cholesterol was 280 and is now down to 170! – KC

Thank you so very much for your food information. I have been religiously following your advice for about two years. I've lost 100 pounds. You literally don't have time to read my long litany of health improvements, but they range from dramatically improved mood to amazing night vision. – BI

For more testimonials see page 240.

Scientific studies show that chronic preventable health conditions, including high blood pressure, high cholesterol, type 2 diabetes, heart disease, and stroke are increasingly being associated with excess weight. For example, experts estimate that one-half of all type 2 diabetes cases could be prevented simply by controlling obesity!

Readers' Stories About Weight Loss and Increased Energy Levels

Many readers commented that the key to losing weight was forgetting about counting calories and focusing instead on eating more of the World's Healthiest Foods. Readers told us that these foods not only helped them feel more vibrant and energetic, but they successfully lost weight without feeling deprived or sacrificing anything—including enjoyment—in the process:

I've been researching and preparing meals based on WHFoods.org for the past month. I feel far more alive, alert, enlightened, and energized. I now experience greater degrees of balance, equilibrium, and sound sleep and no more mood swings.

New Beginnings: I'm a 40+ community college professor who ought to have learned about the World's Healthiest Foods a long time ago. When I stumbled across your web site late last year while searching the Internet for information on wholesome and healthy eating, I could not believe my good fortune.

For virtually all of my adult life I've been trying to lose weight, cut down on fatty foods and eat healthily – but without much success. As I worked my way through the stock of information on your site something clicked on in my brain: This is it! This is the grand design in the nutritional cosmos. This is the way I must go. This is the light among the tunnels of information available on the net.

Your approach to helping people find and lead a healthy lifestyle through eating WHFoods surpasses all that I've ever purchased and read about. Really. Your site is professionally designed and presented so efficiently and appealingly that the readers can easily navigate its portals. You showcase an avalanche of life-saving, healthful information that I use every day, now. What a boon to my generation and the future! And I still can't believe that I have free access to this information all day, every day.

I just had to write to express my delight. I've renounced my high-fat, senseless, cultural eating habits. I've been researching and preparing meals based upon WHFoods for the past month. I feel far more alive, alert, enlightened and energized. I now know that my family will be better nourished and balanced by eating these foods. I never realized that mere foods could affect our health and moods in critical ways. I now experience greater degrees of balance, equilibrium, sound sleep and no more mood swings, in particular. Surprisingly too, the WHFoods (legumes, fruit smoothies, veggie salads & entrees, nuts, brown rice, etc.) I've been preparing have certainly decreased the desire for second helpings because they're so satisfying and fulfilling. All of this is still unbelievable and yet so simple. – Michelle

I have lost weight while I eat more. I have also found more energy and strength. And for that reason, I wish to thank you very much. – Mitch

It has been nearly six months since I began changing over to the World's Healthiest Foods, and I am pleasantly surprised at my increase in energy, the loss of dress sizes, and the overall feeling of good health. I find that my refrigerator is not filled with "empty calories" and that I can always have great snacks and healthy delicious food to eat. – Terri

Thank you!!! I just needed to thank you for changing my life. This information has created a better, healthier, and more energetic me. I have lost close to 30 pounds by changing my way of eating. I was a terrible fast-food, processed-food eater who never drank water or ate any kind of fruit; now I think I would die without those things. Just the thought of fast foods makes me sick. I just couldn't let this change in my life go without thanking you so much for helping me. – DL

Energy is what makes the world go round and our bodies' are no different. We need energy to move our muscles, keep us breathing, keep our heart beating, and maintain our body temperature. Nothing helps to make day-to-day life more enjoyable than an abundance of energy.

Maintaining a healthy metabolism is one key to having plenty of energy. What is metabolism? Metabolism is the complex chemistry that takes place in your body every second to keep you alive and healthy. And a healthy metabolism requires optimal nutritional support—the kind of support you will get from enjoying foods like the World's Healthiest Foods—especially those rich in protein, magnesium, iron, sulfur-containing compounds, and vitamins B1 (thiamin), B2 (riboflavin), B3 (niacin), B5 (pantothenic acid) and B6 (pyridoxine).

For more testimonials see page 240.

Readers' Stories About Healthy Weight Loss and Cooking

Readers have written to me about how much they love the combination of great tasting food and the quick and easy preparation of the World's Healthiest Foods found in our recipes. While many people don't associate cooking with weight loss, when you consider how important the flavor, taste, and enjoyment of food is to your life you can see that they very much go hand-in-hand—how your food is prepared is closely related to your enjoyment of it. My cooking methods and great tasting recipes therefore are the two important factors that make the transition to a lifestyle change of healthy eating easier and more enjoyable:

I started using the Healthy Sauté method of preparing food. I am a 65-year-old male who now weighs 172 pounds. I began at 245 pounds. I only use fresh veggies, fruits, etc. and the Healthy Sauté method for cooking. I do grill and eat meat/fish in moderation. I want to thank you so much for changing my life. I have maintained my current weight for 6 months and increased my exercise regimen from swimming to a full gym program. Food now is so important to me because you have been there to help people like me. Keep up the good work. I love the recipes. I have discovered so much. – DD

With your assistance I have lost 17 pounds, which previously seemed impossible. Your recipes taste so good—easy and fast, which is what we all need. I have purchased your book for my mother, sister and two friends. I share your daily recipes with my co-workers who also want your book. Thanks so much for providing all of us so much help. – Cheryl

I bought George's book, The World's Healthiest Foods, in January and began to look at how I ate, what I ate, how much I ate. After less than four months, I found my weight down almost 20 pounds; my husband (who had not meant to go on a diet, but whose cook is, yes, me) had lost seven pounds as well. My energy level has increased as well, and the level of fruit and veggie intake has increased dramatically. Salads became an adventure, and the use of nuts and spices added zest to the foods. – Ann

Your Plan meets all of my requirements for becoming healthy: simple prep time, quick and easy cooking methods, and gourmet tasting meals every time! I've lost over thirty pounds in three and one-half months. I have more energy than I can use, and better skin than I ever would have thought possible. The World's Healthiest Foods are truly the best guide for those of us who want to pursue health while having time to enjoy life outside of the kitchen. – Rosemary

I am loving this site, and my interest in whole foods and preparing (with your methods of course) my meals has never been like this. – BI

The style of cooking you have perfected makes food preparation so easy and the outcome so richly flavorful. – Marie

I believe healthy weight loss demands two things—eating health-promoting foods and eating foods that taste great. The goal of this book is to make that combination easy for you. As I have said on many an occasion, no matter how nutritious a food, no one will continue to eat it if it doesn't taste good. My new way of cooking and recipes not only retain the nutrients in the foods you prepare but also enhance their flavor so your taste buds don't feel deprived. I can't think of anything more important to support a lifestyle change to healthy eating and healthy weight loss.

Because the sheer pleasure of eating is high on my list of values I have spent years developing innovative ways to prepare the World's Healthiest Foods. Some recipes have been tested over 100 times until I got it right. Based on the Mediterranean-style of eating, which comes from some of the healthiest people in the world, my recipes look exquisite to the eye, taste delicious, and provide you with great nutritional value.

While this book focuses on how to include more World's Healthiest Vegetables in your meals, similar to Mediterranean cuisine, the meals also include fruits, legumes, nuts and seeds, fish, and lean meats. While some of these foods have considerably more calories than vegetables, they are important whole foods that provide you enjoyment and a full range of nutrients. Feeling well satiated with nutritious foods helps you avoid foods that are full of calories and "empty" of nutrition.

Going hand-in-hand with making *World's Healthiest Vegetable* the centerpiece of your meals is cooking them in a way that makes them taste so good you'll eat them because you want to rather than because you "have" to. Preparing more of your meals at home has become increasingly popular not only because it is less expensive, but because it helps improve our health by controlling the amounts of added sugar, salt, and fats in our meals. Reducing the intake of added sugar and fats also helps us lose weight. Research now confirms that people who frequently eat out tend to be heavier than those who eat more of their meals at home. My new way of cooking methods and recipes will help you make in-home cooking quick and easy (most recipes take only 7 minutes). You will prepare food that will not only improve your health but that also tastes great!

For more testimonials see page 240. The Readers' letters were an inspiration to me!

Thanks to Our Readers

I want to express my sincere appreciation to all the Readers who took the time to relay their stories to us. We set out to help people eat healthier and feel better, and along the way, we unexpectedly started getting testimonial after testimonial from people who not only felt better, but who were also losing weight. The people who wrote to us were not necessarily even trying to lose weight. But they did, and in their minds, the World's Healthiest Foods were definitely involved. I don't know why these individuals lost weight. In fact, I know that in most research studies where people try to lose weight by making grocery lists, spending more time in the kitchen, and making all their own decisions about foods and serving sizes, they don't lose weight. But that wasn't the case for the individuals who took the time to write to us. They DID lose weight. How did this happen? What are the most likely explanations? I'd like to share our thoughts with you about some of the reasons I think this might be possible for you.

CHAPTER 2

Why the World's Healthiest Foods are Good for You

The Readers who wrote to us made a lifestyle change to having the *World's Healthiest Foods* as the foundation for a healthier way of eating. So, by now you must be wondering, "What is it about the World's Healthiest Foods that make them so effective in producing vibrant health and energy?"

Because the *World's Healthiest Foods* provide what is essential and leave out what is unnecessary, they are custom-tailored for optimal health. And because you can eat plenty of the World's Healthiest Foods for great nutrition and to help you feel satiated you may be less likely to want to indulge in foods that are nutrient-poor and calorie-rich—a formula that often leads to poor health and weight gain.

The *World's Healthiest Foods* help promote optimal health because they are whole foods that contain all of the nutrients that nature provides to ensure the health and life of plants and animals. When we eat the World's Healthiest Foods, we enjoy those same protective qualities nature has supplied; nothing is contained in these foods that doesn't need to be there. Because the World's Healthiest Foods provide what is essential and leave out what it unnecessary, they are custom-tailored for optimal health.

World's Healthiest Foods Contain Everything You Need

University scientists and public health officials all agree that eating foods like the *World's Healthiest Foods* results in a lower risk of obesity and preventable diseases, while also promoting healthy aging and higher energy levels. Time and again, epidemiological studies—a type of study in which the diet consumed by individuals is compared to their development of preventable diseases over a period of years or decades—show that people who consume these foods have a lower risk of developing obesity, cardiovascular disease (CVD), and arthritis than people whose diets emphasize processed, refined un-whole foods.

So what specifically is it about the World's Healthiest Foods that gives them power and valuable health-promoting effects? Since their value is a reflection of both what they do contain and what they do not contain let's explore both perspectives so that we can fully appreciate how and why these whole foods support well-being and vitality.

Scientific researchers are finding that a higher consumption of these healthy foods is associated with a reduced risk of obesity and early aging. They are now working on understanding exactly why whole foods provide health protection and have identified many compounds present in these foods that appear to be helpful. Among the most researched are vitamins and minerals, antioxidants, phytonutrients, and dietary fibers and resistant starches. They help the body grow, create energy, and maintain its physiological functions as well as help reduce risk of inflammation. They also help people have more energy and vitality, a stronger immune system (catch fewer colds), healthier looking skin, and improvement in memory, while also promoting better heart health.

Vitamins and Minerals

Both vitamins and minerals are essential to human nutrition as they aid in the metabolic functioning of the body. They differ in that vitamins are considered organic compounds (contain carbon in their chemical structure) while minerals in their elemental form are considered inorganic (and contain no carbon). Since the body does not produce most vitamins and minerals, we must get them from the food that we eat. There is a large array of both vitamins and minerals, each playing their own particular role to helping us keep healthy. That's where the World's Healthiest Foods come in. Selecting a variety of nutrient-rich foods concentrated in vitamins and minerals helps keep your body functioning optimally.

Antioxidants

"Antioxidant" has become a common word in nutritional vocabulary, but what actually are antioxidants and why are they so beneficial to our health? Antioxidants are substances that help protect our cells and body parts from oxygen-related damage. There are many different ways in which substances can function as antioxidants. I'd like to give you a much closer look at antioxidants by telling you about one of the most common of these ways.

One important way that a substance can function as an antioxidant is by giving away electrons. Substances in our body become more reactive when they are left with an uneven number of electrons. (Electrons like to exist in pairs and don't like being "unpaired.") Substances with unpaired electrons are called "free radicals." Many different types of events can be involved with free radical formation, including exposure to UV radiation, toxins, and pollutants. Free radicals can even be formed during our cells' own energy-producing processes. One potential danger posed by excessive formation of free radicals is the potential for these free radicals to damage nearby structures in the body, including the wall of a blood vessel or the membrane of a cell. By supplying free radicals with additional electrons, antioxidants can help prevent this potential damage.

However, when antioxidants give away electrons, another problem occurs. The antioxidants themselves become radicals because they now have unpaired electrons. The solution to this problem is for other antioxidants to provide them with the needed electrons. This process of losing and gaining electrons is like a juggling act. As long as you have a lot of different jugglers staying very active and throwing a lot of balls (electrons) back and forth in the air at the same time, your body stays healthy.

It is important that antioxidants work together as a team. It's like they are a juggling team that keeps us healthy as long as the focus is on teamwork. And this teamwork comes from enjoying a wide variety of *World's Healthiest Foods*, all of which provide a diverse spectrum of antioxidants. For example these could include vitamins A, C and E; the trace minerals selenium and zinc; and a variety of important phytonutrients such as flavonoids and carotenoids, all of which can be juggled to provide optimal antioxidant protection.

Phytonutrients

Cultures whose diet primarily features plant-based foods such as fruits, vegetables, whole grains, legumes, and nuts and seeds have been found to have increased longevity and reduced rates of the many preventable diseases so common in populations consuming the standard American diet. Researchers traditionally have attributed the health-promoting effects of plant foods to their comprehensive array of vitamins, minerals, and fiber. More recently, however, research studies are uncovering a new story. Plant foods contain thousands of other compounds in addition to macronutrients (complex carbohydrates, proteins, fats, and fiber) and micronutrients (vitamins and minerals). These many other compounds are collectively known as phytonutrients (*phyto*=plant) such as lycopene in tomatoes, beta-carotene in carrots, and chlorophyll in green vegetables. Simply put, phytonutrients are active compounds in plants that have been shown to provide benefit to humans when consumed.

Phytonutrients serve various functions in plants, helping to protect the plant's vitality. For example, some phytonutrients protect the plant from UV radiation while others protect it from insect attack. Not only do phytonutrients award benefit to the plants but they also provide benefits to those who enjoy plant food. That's because they have health-promoting properties including antioxidant, anti-inflammatory, and liver health-promoting activities.

Fruits and vegetables are concentrated sources of phytonutrients; other plant foods like whole grains, legumes/beans, nuts and seeds, and herbs and spices also contain phytonutrients. Since many phytonutrients also serve as the pigment that gives foods their deep hues, you can identify many phytonutrient-rich foods by looking for colorful foods; for example, look for foods that are blue or purple like blueberries, blackberries, and red cabbage (rich in flavonoids); yellow-orange foods like carrots, winter squash, papaya, and melon (rich in beta-carotene); red or pink foods like tomatoes, guava, and watermelon (rich in lycopene); and green foods like kale, spinach, and collard greens (rich in chlorophyll). Yet, since not all phytonutrients give color, it's important to not overlook some off-white foods as well—for example, garlic, onions, and leeks are rich in powerful sulfur-containing phytonutrients.

The array of phytonutrients offered by plant-based foods further supports the fact that these foods can make important contributions to our health. Although they are officially considered "non-essential nutrients"—meaning that their intake is not necessary for survival—phytonutrients seem to truly be essential for the sustenance of a healthy life, one full of health and abundant energy. Hopefully, one day as the accepted nutrition paradigm changes from foods for their ability to prevent outright deficiencies to foods for their ability help prevent disease and promote longevity, the true importance of these phytonutrients will be recognized.

Dietary Fiber

The *World's Healthiest Fruits, Vegetable, Legumes, Nuts, and Seeds* are rich in health-promoting dietary fiber. Dietary fiber supports healthy digestion by helping regulate the rate that foods moves through the intestines, by helping prevent constipation, by providing support for "friendly" bacteria in the large intestine, and by other means.

Until very recently, the functions of a specific type of fiber were determined by whether or not the fiber was classified as soluble or insoluble. Virtually all fiber-containing foods contain a mixture of soluble and insoluble fibers. However, some foods have a higher proportion of soluble fiber, and others have a higher proportion of insoluble fiber. Foods particularly rich in soluble fiber—including oat bran, beans, peas, lentils, nuts, seeds, psyllium, apples, pears, and strawberries—are known to reduce blood cholesterol levels, normalize blood sugar levels, and lower the risk of heart disease and type 2 diabetes. Food especially rich in insoluble fiber, including whole grains (and particularly some whole grain brans, like wheat bran), brown rice, nuts, seeds, carrots, cucumbers, zucchini, celery, dark leaf vegetables grapes, and tomatoes are known to help promote bowel health Despite the widespread use of the terms "soluble" and "insoluble" to describe the health benefits of dietary fiber, many medical and nutrition experts contend that these terms do not adequately describe the physiological effects of all the different types of fiber.

Studies show that total fiber intake of both kinds can lower risk of heart disease, metabolic syndrome, and obesity. For weight loss, fiber is important because it makes you feel full longer and curbs overeating. High-fiber foods are filling; they require more chewing and stay longer in your stomach, absorbing water, and helping you feel full.

Resistant Starches

Resistant starches are a unique class of carbohydrates, which can pass through the small intestine undigested and then proceed to the large intestine where they can undergo bacterial fermentation. One of the byproducts of resistant starch fermentation can be butyric acid, a short-chain fatty acid that can support the health and healing of cells in the small and large intestine.

What the World's Healthiest Foods Don't Contain is Also Important

In addition to the the *World's Healthiest Foods* containing the nutrients needed to promote optimal health, the other important aspect of enjoying them is what they do not contain. The synergy of beneficial compounds inherent in whole foods—like the *World's Healthiest Foods*—may only be one piece of the puzzle as to why these foods are better for your health than un-whole foods. Whole foods, by their nature, differ from refined foods in that they are not processed with an array of chemical additives or the addition of sugar, salt, and fat. Added sugars and fats are important contributing factors to the obesity epidemic that we are experiencing in the U.S.

What is the Secret of the World's Healthiest Foods and Why They are So Beneficial

The *World's Healthiest Foods* are whole foods whose benefits are, in part, derived from the fact that the nutrients they contain act in concert, rather than simply as single agents. These foods are therefore more than simply the sum of their individual parts. Although researchers have identified and typically focus on single compounds in whole foods that promote health (e.g., vitamins and minerals, antioxidants, phytonutrients, dietary fiber, and resistant starches), and compounds in refined, processed foods that are health detractors (e.g., synthetic chemical additives), this reductionistic focus only tells part of the story of why a diet rich in whole foods provides numerous health benefits.

The beauty of the *World's Healthiest Foods*, and their associated health benefits, seems to be a reflection of the natural synergy of all of their components: the totality of what they provide. This is not to say the benefits of each of the isolated components are not important—they are. It just means we should not lose the forest for the trees that is, in their natural state in whole foods, these compounds work together synergistically. Current scientific research supports this concept. Health-promoting foods work better when consumed containing as much of their original complement of nutrients as as possible. Studies exploring the relationship between diet and health consistently show health benefits from eating minimally processed whole foods, whereas, studies focusing solely on isolated compounds have yielded mixed results.

So, while a food's individual components may be important, research continues to support that our bodies need more than isolated nutrients; for optimal health we need the full complement of nutrients in whole foods. This complement of thousands of health-promoting compounds provides a synergy of health-protecting effects in our bodies and is likely to contain many yet-to-be discovered beneficial components that are also integral to the vibrant health offered from The World's Healthiest Foods.

Optimal Health and the World's Healthiest Foods

Scientific studies have shown that the symphony of health-promoting nutrients in foods such as the World's Healthiest Foods are the key to having your body systems function at their best. This includes your nervous system, cardiovascular system, digestive system, musculoskeletal system, and detoxification system. Having your body systems function at their best also means having a limited amount of stored fat. We now know that fatty tissue is not only a passive storage place for emergency calories, but also a type of tissue that has hormonal function and can have a regulatory effect on our inflammatory system. If we deposit too much fat on our body, we run the risk of increased problems with other body systems, including our inflammatory system.

Can the Foods I Eat Affect My Genes and Make Me Healthier

The foods we eat directly affect the expression of our genes. The nutrients in the foods we consume communicate with our genes, delivering information that alters which aspects of our genes—those that promote health or those that engender dysfunction and disease—will be activated.

Research has now shown that even the genes we've inherited that render us more susceptible to various chronic diseases do not, inevitably, cause disease. Their damaging messages sometimes remain silent unless we make food, lifestyle, or environmental choices that trigger them into action.

In fact, our genes are so responsive to our dietary choices that eating foods that do not provide for our genetically inherited needs is now recognized as a major factor in the development of virtually all chronic degenerative diseases, including cardiovascular disease, type 2 diabetes, arthritis, digestive disorders, loss of mental function, and even many types of cancers.

The good news is that hundreds of recent studies have provided sufficient information so that you can choose a healthy way of eating that is most likely to tell your genes to create your healthiest possible phenotype. The research building on the results of the Human Genome Project has shown that—with the exception of a few traits like eye color and an increased potential risk for some diseases—our genetic inheritance (or genotype) holds a variety of options for what will be expressed and manifested as our actual physical self (our phenotype).

How Fruits, Vegetables, Nuts, Seeds and Whole Grains Talk to Your Genes

Fruits, vegetables, whole grains, nuts, seeds, beans and legumes contain a lot more than carbohydrate, protein, fat, fiber, vitamins and minerals. Each and every type of plant contains thousands of protective compounds called phytonutrients (phyto means plant). Phytonutrients—like flavonoids, catechins, phenols, anthocyanins, isothio-cyanates, carotenoids, terpenoids, and a legion of other compounds with tongue-twisting names—can modify gene expression, each promoting healthy physiological function in a slightly different way.

To get the myriad benefits that occur when phytonutrients communicate with our genes, it's important for us to enjoy lots of whole, unprocessed, organically grown fruits, vegetables, nuts, seeds. and whole grains. The reason that *whole* is important is because many phytonutrients are found in or immediately under a plant's skin (or in the grains, in the outer, fibrous layer). Processing typically removes this phytonutrient-rich outermost layer of plant foods.

For a glimpse into the abundance and complexity of nutrients whole foods deliver, let's look at oranges. When we think "oranges," we think "vitamin C." Yet, as important as this antioxidant is to our health, it's the tip of an orange's nutrient iceberg. Oranges contain more than 170 phytonutrients, including more than 60 bioflavonoids and 20 carotenoids.

And each fruit, vegetable, whole grain, nut, seed, bean, and legume has developed its own unique array of phytonutrients for its personal defense and optimal growth. It's not surprising—given how evolution works—but still a most elegant serendipity that these phytonutrients in plant foods can modify our gene expression in ways that can help pro tect us against premature or unhealthy aging and preventable diseases.

Phytonutrients in whole foods interact with our genes to increase the expression of those that encode for the production of antioxidant and detoxification enzymes, while putting to sleep those that promote inflammation and the development of cancer. In doing so, phytonutrients turn up a host of protective processes in our bodies, while shutting down the damaging ones.

Taking the genetics of healthy eating into consideration the phrase "You are What You Eat" has much larger ramifications than previously believed. If a person is not getting proper nutrients, it shows not only in the individual's mind and body but is also reflected in their genetic expression. On the flip side, a person's overall health and genetic expression can be improved by eating nutrient-rich foods such as the *World's Healthiest Foods.*

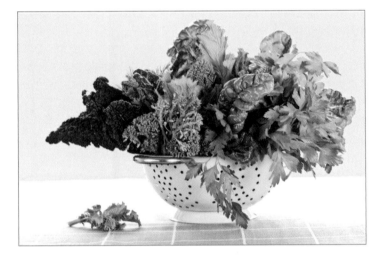

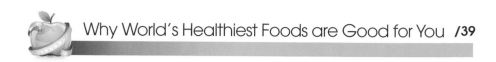

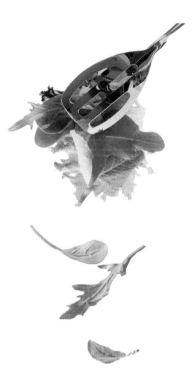

CHAPTER 3

Why Nutrients are Important to Help You Lose Weight and Stay Healthy

Everything we do requires nutrients. Whether we are awake or asleep, exercising or sitting still, we are staying alive with the help of nutrients to support our cells and metabolism. Although some nutrients can be stored in our cells and tissues to a limited degree, many nutrients cannot be stored. Unless we obtain them from food, we simply don't have them! The variety of nutrients we need for optimal nourishment is somewhat staggering: there are vitamins, minerals, proteins, carbohydrates, fats, and literally hundreds of phytonutrients (including carotenoids and flavonoids) that we need to stay optimally healthy.

Nutrient-richness is a measurement of the concentration of nutrients a food can deliver in exchange for the amount of calories it contains.

Nutrient-Rich World's Healthiest Foods =

$$\frac{\textbf{MaximumNutrients}}{\textbf{Minimal Calories}}$$

The classification of a food as nutrient-rich reflects its ability to provide a wealth of nutrients—such as vitamins, minerals, phytonutrients, antioxidants, fiber, amino acids, omega-3 fatty acids, and other

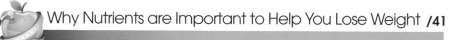

health-promoting compounds—for a minimal amount of calories. (Many researchers use the term "nutrient density" to describe this special dietary combination of high-nutrients plus low-calories.) In sharp contrast, calorie-dense or nutrient-poor foods are ones that provide a small number of nutrients, but a large number of calories; these include processed, refined, and fast foods.

Nutrients and Calories are Important

Since we only have a limited amount of calories that we can consume if we want to achieve optimal health and lose weight, it is essential for us to get as many nutrients as possible in comparison to the number of calories we consume. That's why focusing on the *World's Healthiest Foods* as the centerpiece of your daily meals makes so much sense because they enable you to meet your nutrient needs more easily without exceeding your calorie limits.

Nobody ever – I repeat – EVER lost weight and kept it off while consuming excess calories. ("Excess" in this case, simply means more than the body was able to burn.) In fact, during the weight loss process itself, it is necessary to consume *fewer* calories than your body needs. The goal is to leave your body deprived of some necessary calories so that it will be forced to go into your fat stores and use some of that stored fat as an additional source of calories. Notice that I keep focusing on calories here—not nutrients. You *never* want to leave your body deprived of nutrients! Your body's metabolism cannot function optimally without a rich supply of nutrients, and you need optimal metabolic function to have the best chance at healthy weight loss. So one secret of healthy weight loss is supplying your body with all the nutrients it needs while consuming calories in a lower amount that your body requires.

The Nutrients We Need Each Day

We need hundreds of nutrients to stay healthy and these nutrients must be supplied by the food we eat. Because the *World's Healthiest Foods* provide us with such a wide variety of nutrients, they are a great way to help meet our daily requirements for the nutrients we need each day especially when we are also watching our caloric intake. I'll start first with an overview of some of the nutrients our body needs to achieve optimal health and in the next chapter move on to why the *World's Healthiest Vegetables* are so important to achieving these goals and how to make them taste great so you will enjoy their new role as a prominent feature of your meals.

The following chart contains some well-established and well-researched nutrients that are included in the U.S. Food and Drug Administration's "Reference Values for Nutrition Labeling." It will give you a sense of the variety of some of the nutrients we must get each day from our food if we wish to experience optimal health. Next to each nutrient you'll see the Daily Value (DV) that was established as part of the FDA's labeling program. Please note that this DV value is a population-based goal and is very unlikely to reflect the exact amount of the nutrient that would be best for you (for this information you should seek the advice of a nutrition-oriented healthcare practitioner). Yet, these Daily Values can give you a sense of general nutrient intake goals and how nutrient-rich *World's Healthiest Foods* can provide you with outstanding benefits in terms of Daily Values.

Carbohydrates 300 g	DV*	Minerals	DV*
Protein 50 g		Calcium	1000 mg
Fiber 25 g		Magnesium	320 mg
		Phosphorus	1000 mg
Water Soluble Vitamins		Chloride	3400 mg
Vitamin B1	1.5 mg	Potassium	3500 mg
Vitamin B2	1.7 mg	Sodium	2400 mg
Vitamin B3	20 mg		
Vitamin B5	10 mg	**Trace Minerals**	
Vitamin B6	2 mg	Iron	18 mg
Vitamin B12	6 mcg	Iodine	150 mcg
Folic Acid	400 mcg	Manganese	2 mg
Biotin	300 mcg	Chromium	120 mcg
Vitamin C	60 mg	Zinc	15 mg
		Selenium	70 mcg
Fat Soluble Vitamins		Molybdenum	75 mcg
Vitamin A	5000 IU		
Vitamin D	400 IU	**Essential Fatty Acids**	
Vitamin E	30 IU	Omega-3	2.5g
Vitamin K	80 mcg	Omega-6	12 g

* DV=Daily Value for adults based on 2000 calories a day.

Does the Chart Reflect All the Nutrients We Need?

Please note that this chart is by no means comprehensive; it doesn't show you all of the nutrients you need. For example, many common nutrients—including minerals like **copper** or vitamins like **choline**—have no Daily Value (DV) established for them. Other very important nutrients, like **omega-3 fatty acids**, also have no DV. **Phytonutrients**—plant-derived nutrients including **flavonoids** like quercetin and anthocyanins and catechins)—are also known to be essential to health, but these nutrients have yet to be assigned a DV. And thousands of phytonutrients have yet to be isolated and identified. Yet we know they must exist, because our list of currently known nutrients does not allow us to fully explain all the health benefits we get from whole foods. Since phytonutrients are plant-based nutrients, vegetables are likely to be among the best sources of these yet-to-be identified nutrients.

Nutrients are the Body's Ingredients for Health

Even though most everyone is familiar with the idea of nutrition and nutrients, many people do not really know what nutrients actually *do* and how they work. One of the most important aspects of nutrients is that they rarely work alone; the synergistic interaction between nutrients is what makes them most effective in maintaining optimal health.

It's not as if a nutrient waves a magic wand and voila…a health problem is fixed. The reason that nutrients are related to the prevention of future health problems and the improvement of existing ones is connected to the interaction of nutrients in all of the body's underlying structures and metabolic activities. Nutrients are the resources that our body needs to make and maintain healthy cells. They are the substances that help run our metabolism and allow our body to go about its moment-by-moment physiologic activities. Without them, our body cannot do the things it needs to do: for example, our cells can't communicate, our muscles can't contract, and oxygen can't be carried in our blood.

Those three activities are joined by literally thousands of other activities that go on every second at a metabolic level that is invisible to us but absolutely critical to our health. Nutrients, therefore, are the ingredients in the body's recipe for supporting its underlying structure and function, which serve as the foundation for our physical health. But they do not work independently of each other but synergistically with other nutrients to perform the miracles that sustain life.

You can get a glimpse of the massive underlying health foundation nutrients provide if you take any single nutrient and look at all of the roles it plays in helping to make our bodies function properly. As an example, let's take magnesium.

Magnesium Has Many Health Benefits

Magnesium is a co-factor in over 300 different enzymatic reactions. These include many steps in the energy production cycle as wellas the synthesis of our DNA. Magnesium is also an important component in bone structure and plays an important role in cell-to-cell communication, especially that involving our nerve and muscle cells. Without adequate amounts of magnesium, our bodies wouldn't be able to function properly, which can first lead to lowered energy and then potentially progress to a variety of different signs, symptoms, and health conditions when things aren't working well. As you can also see, it's more complicated than simply saying that the role of magnesium is to promote heart health or bone health, two claims that are often associated with this mineral. Magnesium, like all other nutrients, is needed in hundreds of different ways for support of our underlying metabolic processes, and it is these underlying processes that serve as the true foundation for our overall physical health.

You might think that this more comprehensive and holistic view of health and nutrients would make nourishment more complicated. But it can actually be just the opposite if you select the right kind of foods like the *World's Healthiest Foods*. That's because the *World's Healthiest Foods* are comprehensive and holistic as well! If you consider the *World's Healthiest Foods* as a group, you will discover that their nutrients support every aspect of our metabolic and cellular needs. Not only do they maintain this massive underlying biochemical structure that supports all of our health, but they do so in an optimal way by combining nutrients in their most natural patterns. No supplement will ever be able to achieve this amazing level of synergy between nutrients! All you have to do is focus on enjoying the *World's Healthiest Foods* since their nutrient-richness and natural synergy of nutrients will do the rest of the work for you.

The Orchestra of Nutrients Important for Bone Health

The functioning of calcium for healthy bones will give you another good example of how nutrients don't work independently:

You've no doubt heard that calcium is important for healthy bones. And you may also have heard that osteoporosis—a bone problem that affects 20 million adults in the U.S.—can be "prevented by calcium."

I wish things were this simple! But unfortunately, they are not. Even though calcium plays a pivotal role in maintaining our bone health, it's just not true that calcium, by itself, can prevent the occurrence of osteoporosis.

First of all, there are many more nutrients that bones need to build their structure and density. For example, for good bone health you need magnesium, manganese, zinc, vitamin D, vitamin C, vitamin K, boron, silicon, potassium, and a variety of other nutrients. As you can see, bone health is achieved from a much broader array of nutrients than just calcium. These nutrients are best provided by nutrient-rich foods like the *World's Healthiest Foods*.

Most people are used to thinking about nutrients in a "this cures that" type of way. This way of thinking is sometimes encouraged by the overly simplified positioning of dietary supplements in the marketplace. Manufacturers often include health claims on their product labels that present relatively simple cause-effect relationships between nutrients and health. For example, a supplement manufacturer might claim that calcium builds strong bones, or that fiber maintains bowel regularity, or that vitamin E supports heart health. While all of these connections between nutrients and health have science-based validity, consumers might end up concluding that all they need for a healthy heart is vitamin E, or that nothing more is needed for building strong bones than calcium. The truth

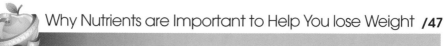

of the matter is that no single nutrient is a magic bullet that can singlehandedly prevent a disease or protect an entire body system like blood vessels or bones.

Just as all of the nutrients that work to perform the miracle of maintaining our health are not yet identified, how the specific interactions of nutrients work for optimal health are not completely understood. But what we do know is that these nutrients and their interactions are essential, and that the only place we get them is from the food we eat.

Total Nutrient-Richness Chart

On the World's Healthiest Foods website (www.WHFoods.org) and in my book, *The World's Healthiest Foods: Essential Guide for the Healthiest Way of Eating,* nutrient-richness is displayed qualitatively. With each World's Healthiest Foods—whether on its webpage or in its dedicated chapter—a Ratings Chart is presented. This Chart shows which of the nutrients the food is a good, very good, or excellent source.

In this book I also include a notation of the quantitative value of a food's nutrient-richness by showing numerical scores that a food achieves in association with each particular nutrient in which it is especially concentrated. I've presented a Total Nutrient-Richness Chart below, which shows the nutrient-richness values of each of these foods. The Total Nutrient-Richness Chart shows the World's Healthiest Foods arranged by food group and total nutrient-richness score. This score was calculated by evaluating each food and seeing how many health-promoting nutrients it provided at a richness level of excellent, very good, or good. You can easily see that vegetables are among the most nutrient-rich foods around. For more details on how this total score was calculated, see page 237 in Appendix 1.

TOTAL NUTRIENT-RICHNESS CHART

Vegetables			Fruits	
Spinach	67		Raspberries	19
Asparagus	57		Strawberries	18
Swiss Chard	53		Cantaloupe	17
Collard Greens	46		Papaya	15
Crimini Mushrooms	43		Pineapple	13
Broccoli	39		Oranges	11
Kale/Mustard Greens	38		Grapes/Raisins	10
Green Beans	37		Apricots	9
Romaine lettuce/salads	34		Grapefruit	9
Brussels Sprouts	34		Blueberries	9
Tomatoes	33		Cranberries	9
Summer Squash	33		Watermelon	8
Cauliflower	33		Kiwi fruit	6
Bell Peppers	31		Bananas	6
Shiitake Mushrooms	28		Plums/Prunes	6
Green Peas	25		Lemons/Limes	4
Celery/Fennel	24		Pears	4
Winter Squash	22		Figs	3
Carrots	21		Apples	2
Cabbage	20		**Fish and Shellfish**	
Eggplant	20		Salmon	25
Beet/Beet Greens	17		Tuna	24
Garlic	15		Sardines	22
Sea Vegetables	15		Shrimp	21
Sweet Potatoes	14		Cod	20
Cucumbers	12		Scallops	14
Onions/Leeks	10		**Nuts and Seeds**	
Avocados	7		Flaxseeds	14
Potatoes	6		Sesame Seeds	13
Corn	5		Pumpkin Seeds	12
Olives/Olive Oil	3		Sunflower Seeds	11
			Almonds	9
			Walnuts	7
			Peanuts	6
			Cashews	6

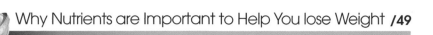

Poultry and Lean Meats			Herbs and Spices	
Calf's Liver	38		Parsley	14
Venison	19		Basil	11
Turkey	16		Turmeric	11
Chicken	14		Cayenne/Red Chili Pepper	11
Lamb	12		Mustard Seeds	10
Beef	9		Cinnamon	10
Beans and Legumes			Black Pepper	10
Dried Peas	25		Dill	6
Soybeans	21		Ginger	5
Lentils	20		Cilantro	3
Kidney Beans/Pinto Beans	19		Rosemary	3
Tofu	19			
Lima Beans	19			
Black Beans/Navy Beans	16			
Garbanzo Beans	16			
Dairy and Eggs				
Yogurt	15			
Eggs	14			
Milk	13			
Cheese	9			
Goat's Milk	9			
Whole Grains				
Oats	8			
Brown Rice	7			
Whole Wheat	7			
Rye	6			
Quinoa	6			
Buckwheat	6			

CHAPTER 4

Why Vegetables Are One-of-a-Kind Foods for Health and Helping You Lose Weight

"We seldom stop to think about what makes the *World's Healthiest Vegetables* (see page 55) so important, or why we need so many each day. The truth about the *World's Healthiest Vegetables* is actually surprising!

How the World's Healthiest Vegetables Help Us Stay Healthy

What's so amazing about the *World's Healthiest Vegetables* is their ability to provide us with such a great variety of nutrients for such few calories. It's not unusual for a *World's Healthiest Vegetable* to provide us with several hundred phytonutrients while costing us under 10 calories per weighted ounce! The amazing nutrient diversity and low-calorie nature of the *World's Healthiest Vegetables* is what makes them altogether unique in a weight loss plan.

The *World's Healthiest Vegetables* are not only some of the most nutrient-rich foods but they bring with them other benefits that may be helpful with weight loss. When people "diet" to try to lose weight, they often find themselves feeling deprived of pleasures related to eating. For example, if you are trying to lose weight and you are restricting yourself to a very small amount of food, you may find yourself really missing the pleasure of chewing. Or to take another example: if you are trying to lose weight and you are relying on a lot of pre-packaged, processed foods, you may find yourself missing the fiber that's needed to help slow down your digestion rate and allow events in your digestive tract to help contribute to your sense of satisfaction. In both situations, the *World's Healthiest Vegetables* may be able to help! The *World's Healthiest Vegetables* are concentrated sources of fiber and give you a great opportunity to take pleasure in chewing.

This is not to say foods other than the *World's Healthiest Vegetables* can't play a very important role in a healthy diet, even a healthy diet geared towards losing weight. All of the *World's Healthiest Foods* can. It's just that their role should be more limited than that of the *World's Healthiest Vegetables*, as their rich concentration of health-promoting nutrients coupled with their low level of calories makes them the perfect food to be the foundation of achieving optimal health and weight loss. The need to emphasize vegetables in a *World's Healthiest Foods'* approach to weight loss cannot be overstated!

Vegetables provide us with an unprecedented array of nutrients. As startling as it might sound, there is no essential nutrient missing from vegetables as a group! Protein, fiber-rich carbohydrates, essential fats, minerals, and vitamins are plentiful in the world of vegetables. And so are phytonutrients, health-supporting compounds found only in plant foods. Researchers estimate that 10,000 or more phytonutrients in vegetables will someday be cataloged and understood. Dozens of health-supportive phytonutrients—featuring antioxidant, anti-inflammatory, and other properties—have already been identified in all commonly eaten vegetables. Sometimes these one-of-a-kind nutrients have even been named after the vegetables themselves; spinasaponins in spinach and celerin in celery are great examples.

The list of nutrients packed inside the *World's Healthiest Vegetables* includes antioxidants like vitamin C and beta-carotene that play such a key role in immune support and in protection of cells and blood vessels. Also included in concentrated amounts are B-complex vitamins like vitamin B6, biotin, and folate. These B-complex vitamins are essential for energy production, proper formation of red blood cells, and healthy nervous system function. Amply supplied by the green leafy vegetables are minerals like calcium and potassium that are essential for healthy blood pressure. And alongside of these vitamins and minerals are abundant amounts of nutrients like fiber, which help regulate digestion, stabilize blood sugars, and facilitate weight management. Because many of the above nutrients are not stored in the body in appreciable amounts, and because vegetables aid in the process of digestion, foods in this remarkable group need to be consumed in generous amounts on a daily basis.

You actually have to hunt in order to find nutrients that are very difficult to obtain in ample amounts from the *World's Healthiest Vegetables.* There are a few, though. As it turns out, the *World's Healthiest Vegetables* are not the best food group for getting omega-3 fatty acids (cold-water fish and nuts are much better), or for certain amino acids (nuts and seeds are much better for sulfur-containing amino acids and dairy products are much better for some of the branched chain amino acids). That's why our *Calorie-Lowering Plan* includes these foods to help create menus that are as balanced for nutrients as possible.

Vegetables, Along with Fruits, Provide a Greater Variety of Phytonutrients Than Any Other Food Group

Vegetables, along with fruits, are at the forefront in helping people to stay healthy because they are the most concentrated sources of health-promoting phytonutrients. Phytonutrients are the compounds that not only provide vegetables with their intense colors but also help protect them as they grow and mature. Examples of phytonutrient groups include anthocyanins—which can be found in red and purple vegetables such as beets and red cabbage—and carotenoids—which can be found in yellow, orange, and red vegetables such as carrots, tomatoes, and winter squash. Chlorophyll is a type of phytonutrient that provide plants, such as kale and Swiss chard, with their bright green color.

These phytonutrients, as well as others found in vegetables (including the *World's Healthiest Vegetables*), help protect your health, just as

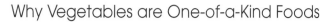

they help protect the plants themselves. The different types of phyto-nutrients work together to help provide antioxidant protection from cellular damage in the body's cardiovascular, immune, respiratory, and central nervous systems. The more *World's Healthiest Vegetables* you eat, the more phytonutrients you will consume, and the more you are likely to benefit from their health-protective properties.

Lutein, beta-carotene, and lycopene are just a few of the phytonutri-ents that researchers are now discovering to have numerous health benefits. Today, the cruciferous vegetables (broccoli, cauliflower, cab-bage, kale, collard greens, mustard greens, and Brussels sprouts) and the allium family of vegetables (onions, garlic, and leeks) are among the *World's Healthiest Vegetables* most studied for their phytonutrient content. All of these *World's Healthiest Vegetables* are known for their health-promoting sulfur compounds, which have been found to reduce the risk of heart disease and the risk of some cancers.

Most of the World's Healthiest Vegetables Can Provide Anti-Inflammatory Benefits

Risk of many chronic diseases—including obesity, diabetes, and heart disease—has been associated with chronic, excessive inflam-mation. Although inflammation is a natural part of our body de-fenses (for example, our body's response to injury or infection), inflammation can be unhealthy if it becomes constant or excessive. Chronic inflammation can happen for many reasons, but overcon-sumption of certain types of food can definitely be a factor in chronic, unwanted inflammation. For example, too great of an intake of hydrogenated oils (potentially containing large amounts of satu-rated fat and trans fat) has been linked to unwanted inflammation. But in the same way that certain foods can increase our risk of un-wanted inflammation, other foods can decrease this risk. Vegetables are high up on the list of foods that have the potential to provide us with anti-inflammatory benefits. For more on inflammation, see page 184.

Most of the vegetables on our list of *World's Healthiest Foods* have shown strong potential in this anti-inflammatory category. These include:

Bell peppers	Cauliflower	Swiss chard
Collard greens	Fennel	Garlic
Broccoli	Fennel	Onions
Cabbage	Green beans	Kale

How the World's Healthiest Vegetables Can Promote Healthy Weight Management

When it comes to helping promote weight loss the low-cal, nutrient-richness of the *World's Healthiest Vegetables* is what makes them unique among all food groups. No food group—not even fruits—can live up to the low-cal, nutrient-richness of vegetables. It's not an exaggeration to say that vegetables, including the *World's Healthiest Vegetables*, are indispensable for optimal nourishment while trying to lose weight!

Of course, if we could eat all day long—and to our heart's content—and not have to worry about gaining weight and becoming obese, our nutrient requirements might not be such a big deal. But overeating is a potential problem for all of us, and for some of us, a real struggle at times. For this reason, eating can sometimes feel like a puzzle: there are so many nutrients we need to enjoy full health, but how are we supposed to get all of these nutrients without overeating and becoming overweight?

It is impossible for us to solve this puzzle without turning to vegetables—and that is why generous daily amounts of the *World's Healthiest Vegetables* are so essential! I analyzed hundreds of foods and those with the lowest calories were vegetables not including starchy vegetables such as corn, potatoes, peas, squashes, and yams. Especially when it comes to the non-starchy vegetables overeating is just not a legitimate concern. The vast majority the *World's Healthiest Vegetables* give us 50 calories per cup (or less) in raw form so you can eat as much as you want with little concern about calories. Here are some examples:

World's Healthiest Vegetables
(foods followed by calories per cup except garlic)

Romaine lettuce – 8	Tomatoes – 32
Cucumbers – 16	Swiss chard* – 35
Celery – 16	Kale *– 36
Cabbage – 18	Brussels sprouts – 38
Summer squash – 18	Spinach* – 41
Eggplant – 20	Garlic (1 oz) – 42
Cauliflower – 27	Collard Greens* – 49
Asparagus – 27	Carrots – 50
Bell peppers – 29	Leeks - 54
Green beans – 31	Beets – 58
Broccoli – 31	Onions – 64
Crimini Mushrooms– 31	

* Note: all vegetables are raw except for those designated by an * which are cooked.

The USDA's traditional food pyramid of dietary recommentions changed in 2011 to the new "MyPlate." Using evidence-based guidelines, MyPlate is especially emphatic about the need to eat more vegetables. In their new graphic, the biggest portion of the plate is dedicated to vegetables!

Just how low is 50 calories per cup? Let's start by comparing the *World's Healthiest Vegetables* to their closest runners-up—namely, fruits. Watermelon will get us down to 49 calories per cup, but only because of its extremely watery nature. With cantaloupe, we're already up to 60 calories, and with berries, our calories-per-cup go start in the 60s and up into the 80s. A cup of juice (like orange juice) takes us up over 100 calories, and a cup of dried fruit (like raisins) gets us close to 450!

Let's compare the *World's Healthiest Vegetables* with foods from a few other food groups to see the calorie difference. With legumes, calories-per-cup fall into the 225-250 range. With nuts and seeds, we're almost always looking at 750 calories or more. As you can see, overeating (in terms of calories) is far less likely with the *World's Healthiest Vegetables*.

Let's take a closer look at another food group that can bring major nutritional benefits to a diet—namely, the whole grains. Virtually all public health organizations recommend daily intake of whole grains, and the U.S. population would definitely reap major health benefits if all refined grains in the average U.S. diet were replaced by 100% whole grains. Whole grains are a good thing! But let's see what happens if we take 8 servings of some very familiar vegetables, and we compare those 8 servings nutritionally to 8 servings of 100% whole grains. In this comparison, we will take 1 serving for each of the following *World's Healthiest Vegetables*—romaine lettuce, spinach, broccoli, tomato, bell pepper, carrot, celery, and onion—and compare the results to 2 servings each of whole wheat, whole grain brown rice, whole oats, and whole cornmeal.

	8 Servings of	8 Servings of
	Whole Vegetables*	Grains**
Calories	177	676

* One serving each for all 8 *World's Healthiest Vegetables* listed above
** Two servings each for all 4 grains listed above

As you can see in the table above, the calorie difference between 8 servings of fresh *World's Healthiest Vegetables* and 8 servings of whole grains is not only substantial (499 calories!) but also of great practical importance in a daily diet. Most of us do not have room to fit 500 extra calories in a day. In fact, if we eat 500 calories more than we need on a daily basis, we are likely to gain about 1 pound of added fat each week or 50 pounds over the year. Yet, despite their much lower calorie content, these 8 servings of vegetables provide

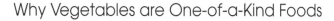
about 50% more nutrients in amounts of 25% of the DV or higher) when compared to the whole grain servings. These nutrients include vitamins B1, B2, B3, B6, E, C, and K; folate; the minerals calcium, magnesium, manganese, molybdenum, phosphorus, and potassium; protein; and fiber. They also provide a greater number of nutrients that offer 100% DV amounts (or greater). Here the nutrients include folate, vitamin K, manganese, and fiber.

When making this comparison between fresh *World's Healthiest Vegetables* and whole grains, it is important to remember that whole grains are not an unhealthy food group or inappropriate in a diet. In fact, on a bite-for-bite basis, the whole grains in our comparison provided greater amounts of vitamin B1, vitamin B5, selenium, and zinc than the fresh vegetables. My point here is to recognize, however, that whole grains provide these greater amounts of these key nutrients at a greater cost in calories as well. From my perspective, this disadvantage in terms of calories makes whole grains a less appropriate focus in weight management than fresh *World's Healthiest Vegetables*. While a healthy diet depends on all key food groups for balanced nourish-ment, successful weight management means special attention to calories, and if we want to keep our nutrient intake high and our calories low, we are much better served by increasing vegetables versus whole grains.

The World's Healthiest Vegetables and Salads—Eat As Much as You Like With No Limit

We need to eat an abundance of the *World's Healthiest Vegetables* and salads every day because they supply an incredible amount of health-promoting nutrients and relatively few calories. Eating the recommended servings of vegetables each day helps promote optimal health. Yet not all vegetables are created equal when it comes to nutrition, calories, or healthy weight loss. So when I recommend a limitless amount of vegetables as part of your new healthy lifestyle, I do not include starchy vegetables, such as potatoes, as part of that formula. Potatoes are the number one vegetable consumed in the U.S. because even French fries are counted as a serving of vegetables. I think that says volumes about the health and weight problem facing our nation today.

Our bodies are very adaptive and can obviously survive on less than the recommended amounts of vegetables each day, but over the long run, inadequate intake of vegetables is likely to cost most U.S. adults a substantial price in terms of health. Negative effects may be subtle and go unnoticed for awhile as they may take a long time to fully develop. However, they can't be avoided; without adequate servings of vegetables, most people in the U.S. would have too much difficulty finding alternative sources of the nutrients necessary for good health. That list of necessary nutrients includes vitamins, minerals, dietary fiber, and literally thousands of protective phytonutrients, the importance of which are just now being revealed in the scientific research. It's important to remember that lack of adequate vegetable consumption has been associated with problems in our body systems like our digestive system and immune system, and also with increased risk for many types of preventable diseases. Eating plenty of the *World's Healthiest Vegetables* every day can also help increase energy levels, improve memory, prevent colds and flu, support healthier skin, reduce risk of heart disease, and help maintain optimal health.

Examples of the World's Healthiest Vegetables

Spinach

To further explain the unique qualities of nutrient-rich World's Healthiest Vegetables, and to clearly illustrate how important they are to health, I want to share with you some food comparisons. Following is a chart showing the contributions of nutrients, including the % Daily Value (DV) for nutrients To further explain the unique qualities of nutrient-rich World's Healthiest Vegetables, and to clearly illustrate how important they are to health, I want to share with you some food comparisons. Following is a chart showing the contributions of nutrients, including the % Daily Value (DV) for nutrients of which spinach is a concentrated source.

1 cup cooked spinach Nutrient	DV (%)	41 calories Nutrient	DV (%)
vitamin K	1110.6	vitamin B6 (pyrodoxine)	22.0
vitamin A	377.3	tryptophan	21.9
manganese	84.0	vitamin E	18.7
folate	65.7	dietary fiber	17.3
magnesium	39.1	copper	15.5
iron	35.7	vitamin B1 (thiamin)	11.3
vitamin C	29.4	protein	10.7
vitamin B2 (riboflavin)	24.7	phosophorus	10.1
calcium	24.5	zinc	9.1
potassium	24.0	omega 3 fatty acids	7.1

(Lutein/zeaxanthin are carotenoids that are also highly concentrated in spinach. Since there is not a DV for carotenoids, however, they are not included above.)

As you can see, one cup of cooked spinach contains only 41 calories. That's 2.3% of the calories that would be included in a 2,000 calorie diet. Yet, for just over 2% of your daily calories, you get between 10% and 100% of the DailJ137 Value for 18 nutrients! In addition to these remarkable benefits for these nutrients, this one-cup serving of spinach lets you exceed (by leaps and bounds) your daily intake goals for vitamin K (1111%) and pro-vitamin A (377%). All of these amazing benefits and—if you were aiming for 1500 daily calories— you still have about 1459 calories left to enjoy and "use" to get more nutrients! That's almost 98% of your day's calories left to enjoy.

Cruciferous Vegetables

In terms of conventional nutrients (vitamins, minerals, proteins, carbs, and fats), I cannot find another vegetable group that is as high in vitamin A carotenoids, vitamin C, folic acid, and fiber as the cruciferous vegetables (broccoli, cauliflower, kale, collard greens, Brussels sprouts, cabbage, and bok choy). As a group, the cruciferous vegetables are simply superstars in these conventional nutrient areas. The astonishing concentration of vitamin A carotenoids in cruciferous vegetables and their unusually high content of vitamin C and manganese are clearly key components in their growing reputation as an antioxidant vegetable group. And 100 calories' worth of cruciferous vegetables (about 5–6% of a daily diet's caloric intake) provides about 25–40% of your daily fiber requirement! As impressive as they are in terms of their conventional nutrient content, cruciferous vegetables are even more renowned for their sulfur-containing phytonutrients. At a minimum, I recommend including cruciferous vegetables as part of your diet 2–3 times per week, and make the serving size at least $1^1/_2$ cups.

Now, I'd like to tell you more about some specific cruciferous vegetables.

Kale

Tuscan or Lacinato Kale is one of the favorite varieties of kale, which is becoming recognized as a rising star when it comes to health-promoting vegetables. Kale is a member of the cruciferous family of vegetables and one of the most nutrient-rich vegetables around. While not as familiar to many people as broccoli, I have discovered that when I introduce friends to kale, it becomes one of their favorite vegetables. Along with providing an excellent source of vitamins A, K, and C, researchers now identify over 45 different flavonoids in kale. These phytonutrients may account for their many health-promoting properties, including lowering cholesterol and encouraging detoxification. Kale is also rich in dietary fiber, which may help you feel satiated.

1 cup cooked kale Nutrient	DV (%)	36 calories Nutrient	DV (%)
vitamin K	1327.6	iron	6.5
vitamin A	354.1	magnesium	5.8
vitamin C	88.8	vitamin E	5.6
manganese	27.0	omega 3 fatty acids	5.4
dietary fiber	10.4	vitamin B2 (riboflavin)	5.3
copper	10.0	protein	4.9
trypotophan	9.4	vitamin B1 (thiamin)	4.7
calcium	9.4	folate	4.2
vitamin B6 (pyrodoxine)	9.0	phosphorus	3.6
potassium	8.5	vitamin B3 (niacin)	3.2

Broccoli

Broccoli is one of America's favorite vegetables and is a member of the family of cruciferous vegetables. It provides you with a wealth of vitamins A and C, bone-building vitamin K, and health-promoting phytonutrients. It also has plenty of fiber, which can help you feel full—a feeling that can be very welcomed when you are trying to lose weight.

1 cup raw broccoli Nutrient	DV (%)	31 calories Nutrient	DV (%)
vitamin C	135.3	vitamin B2 (riboflavain)	6.5
vitamin K	115.6	phosphorus	6.0
vitamin A	11.3	pantothenic acid	5.2
folate	14.3	protein	5.1
dietary fiber	9.5	magnesium	4.8
manganese	9.5	calcium	4.3
tryptophan	9.4	vitamin B1 (thiamin)	4.0
potassium	8.2	iron	3.7
vitamin B6 (pyrodoxine)	8.0	vitamin E	3.5

Cabbage

While green cabbage is the most commonly eaten variety, I highly recommend trying red cabbage because of its added nutritional benefits and its robust hearty flavor. The rich red color of red cabbage reflects it concentration of anthocyanin polyphenols, which contribute to red cabbage containing significantly more protective phytonutrients than green cabbage. Interest in anthocyanin pigments continues to intensify because of their health benefits as dietary antioxidants, as an anti-inflammatory, and their potentially protective, preventative, and therapeutic roles in a number of human diseases.

1 cup raw cabbage Nutrient	DV (%)	18 calories Nutrient	DV (%)
vitamin K	66.5	folate	7.5
vitamin C	42.7	vitamin B6 (pyrodoxine)	4.5
dietary fiber	7.0	potassium	3.4
manganese	5.5	tryptophan	3.1

Salads for Nutrients and Calorie Control

Most people who struggle with getting 5-9 daily servings of vegetables forget that enjoying a salad—as part of lunch and/or dinner—can put them well on their way to meeting these goals. That's because a food like romaine lettuce is more than just a base for a delicious salad. It provides an impressive handful of nutrients for an equally impressive small number of calories (you can have 10 servings of salad greens for less than 100 calories). If you look at the chart below, you'll see how two cups of romaine lettuce—the least you'd probably use for making a salad—is so nutrient-rich. For just 16 calories, you're well on your way to meeting your daily goals for vitamin K, pro-vitamin A, vitamin C, folate, manganese, and chromium, while also enjoying a host of other health-promoting nutrients. This is why I recommend eating a salad made of romaine lettuce (or another type of nutrient-rich lettuce) everyday. Some other popular varieties of lettuce include (foods follwed by calories per cup):

Arugula 5

Baby spinach 7

Butterhead 7

Boston, Bibb 7

Endive 7

Mixed salad 9

Leaf lettuce (green or red) 10

Water cress 10

2 cups romaine Nutrient	DV (%)	16 calories Nutrient	DV (%)
vitamin K	120.4	molybdenum	7.5
vitamin A	163.7	potassium	6.6
vitamin C	37.6	iron	5.1
folate	32.0	vitamin B1 (thiamin)	4.7
dietary fiber	7.9	vitamin B2 (riboflavin)	3.5

(Beta-carotene and lutein/zeaxanthin are carotenoids that are also found in concentrated amounts in romaine lettuce. Since there is not a DV for carotenoids, they are not included above.)

CHAPTER 5

Why Weight Loss Without Dieting Is Good For You

Usually when you embark on a weight loss diet, it means giving up the pleasure of eating! Weight loss diets often require letting others make all the decisions for us, and they usually involve having to give up the joys of eating for a promise that we will lose weight.

Many weight loss diets ask us to turn our lives completely over to a pre-determined script not of our making. We are often asked to build our breakfasts, lunches, and dinners around highly processed foods that we didn't select, cook, or even choose from a list of our favorites. By letting someone else make all of these decisions for us, we give up the joys of eating for a promise that we will lose weight.

Most weight loss plans require you to follow some new type of diet for the first time in your life. These weight loss plans depend upon a certain amount of novelty. They are betting that you've never eaten this way before (and chances are, you will never eat this way again!). They are also assuming that you aren't familiar with the "special twists" in their theory of weight loss. They give you a diet that includes these special twists in the hope that you'll find it new and interesting enough to make you willing to put up with whatever unbalanced regimen is prescribed through a period of initial weight loss.

I personally found that when I changed to eating more of the *World's Healthiest Foods*, I became more in touch with the foods that my body needed. I craved and relied less and less on the sweet, fat, and salty foods that were so convenient to satisfy my hunger. I was so much more satisfied that I didn't really desire the nutrient-poor foods. As some of our Readers had shared with us, they also had similar experiences.

Being "Diet-Free" Lets You Enjoy Whole, Unprocessed, Nutrient-Rich Foods

In any diet plan—including any weight loss plan—it's important to nourish yourself with nutrients rather than just fueling yourself with calories. Nourishing yourself with nutrients might mean eating more of certain foods—not less! And that's exactly the approach that I've taken. My approach does not focus on eating less but on eating more—more unprocessed, whole, nutrient-rich foods that are low in calories, that taste great, and that can help you feel full and satisfied. And of all the *World's Healthiest Foods,* the *World's Healthiest Vegetables* are the best choice to help meet that goal.

What makes the *World's Healthiest Foods* (and especially the *World's Healthiest Vegetables*) beneficial to health is not just that they are rich in one or two specific nutrients but because they contain a whole range of nutrients that work together to provide greater health benefits than those working alone. What that means is that there is no one miracle food or miracle nutrient. There is only the miracle of how the different aspects of a variety of nutrients work together to provide you with optimal health. Selecting nutrient-rich foods that are the lowest in calories makes a great foundation for potential weight loss.

Enjoy Foods Low in Calories That Taste Great

When you are trying to lose weight, you are very likely to want some low-calorie foods in your diet. You might be able to construct a nutritionally adequate weight loss diet that contains mostly high-calorie foods, but such a diet is very likely to leave you dissatisfied because you will not get enough food volume. There is no better example of foods that can be enjoyed in high volume due to their low calorie content than the *World's Healthiest Vegetables.* The *World's Healthiest Vegetables* are not only among the lowest calorie foods in the world but they can also help you feel satisfied—one of the keys to helping prevent overeating. As you can see in the chart on page 55 the low calorie count for the *World's Healthiest Vegetables* speaks for themselves.

In the previous chapter I talked about the many health-promoting properties of the *World's Healthiest Vegetables*. My intent in this chapter is not only to help you with a conceptual understanding of why the *World's Healthiest Vegetables* can be so valuable for health and weight loss but perhaps more importantly to provide you with practical ways to make them taste great. This way including more of the *World's Healthiest Vegetables* into your new healthier eating lifestyle is fun and enjoyable. That's why I want to share with you the ways I select, store, prepare, and cook the *World's Healthiest Vegetables.*

Easy Tips for Best Enjoyment of the World's Healthiest Vegetables

When it comes to retaining nutritional value, flavor, and visual appeal, the *World's Healthiest Vegetables* require special care and attention because they are delicate in nature. Properly selecting, storing, preparing, and cooking *World's Healthiest Vegetables* (if they are to be cooked) are all important aspects of retaining their health-promoting benefits, as well as their flavor.

Selecting Fresh Nutrient-Rich World's Healthiest Vegetables

We all like to select the freshest, most nutrient-rich *World's Healthiest Vegetables* possible, which means they are vibrant in color and are not beginning to yellow or becoming limp. Farmers' markets are great places to find locally grown *World's Healthiest Vegetables* in season that are both fresh and less expensive. I also suggest selecting organically grown vegetables, whenever possible, to avoid the pesticide residues that can often be found on conventionally grown produce.

When I am unable to purchase all organically grown produce because of cost or availability I am aided by two lists developed by the

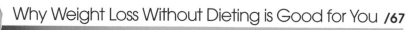

Environmental Working Group to help me determine which ones I want to be sure are organic and which of the conventionally grown ones are safer in terms of pesticide residues.

Each year the Environmental Working Group identifies produce in the U.S. conventional, non-organic food supply that contain the highest number of pesticide residues. The worst offenders have been nicknamed the "Dirty Dozen." The new report issued in 2011 features the following fruits and vegetables as the "Dirty Dozen." They are presented in descending order in terms of the level of pesticide residues, with the one at the top having the most:

- Apples
- Celery
- Strawberries
- Peaches
- Spinach
- Nectarines-imported
- Grapes-imported
- Sweet bell peppers
- Potatoes
- Blueberries-domestic
- Lettuce
- Kale/collard greens

In addition to the "Dirty Dozen" the Environmental Working Group compiles a list of produce that contains the least amount of pesticides. These have come to be known as the "Clean 15, and for 2011 they include:

- Onions
- Sweet corn
- Pineapples
- Avocado
- Asparagus
- Sweet peas
- Mangoes
- Eggplant
- Cantaloupe domestic
- Kiwifruit
- Cabbage
- Watermelon
- Sweet potatoes
- Grapefruit
- Mushrooms

Proper Storage

Did you know you could lose up to 30% of the nutrients in the *World's Healthiest Vegetables* if they are not stored properly? Many factors can contribute to spoilage in *World's Healthiest Vegetables*, including respiration rate (the faster the respiration rate, the more quickly a vegetable will spoil), temperature, humidity, and amount of light. Most *World's Healthiest Vegetables* do best stored in the refrigerator. Exceptions are onions, garlic, and tomatoes (the latter until they become very ripe).

Cleaning Produce

All vegetables, including organically grown vegetables, should be cleaned before cooking or eating raw by rinsing under cold water. This helps them to retain their nutritional value better than some other cleaning methods such as soaking for long periods of time (which can result in loss of nutrients, such as certain water-soluble vitamins). The one exception to rinsing is mushrooms, which I prefer to wipe with a damp paper towel to prevent them from becoming soggy.

Preparation Tips

Cutting or slicing the *World's Healthiest Vegetables* into small pieces also helps them to cook more quickly and evenly, which is important when we want to keep the cooking time to a minimum. Cutting and letting cruciferous vegetables sit for several minutes before cooking can even help enhance their health-promoting benefits. See individual recipes for preparation tips for cruciferous and allium (onions and garlic) vegetables.

Healthy Cooking

Healthy cooking can soften the fibers of the *World's Healthiest Vegetables* and make them easier for many people to digest. This process may help increase the availability of some nutrients to be absorbed. The secret to proper cooking of the *World's Healthiest Vegetables* is twofold: low temperatures and short cooking times.

Healthy cooking brings out the flavor and color of your *World's Healthiest Vegetables* but always in a way that helps to minimize loss of nutrients in comparison to other cooking methods.

The overcooking of vegetables—and their becoming mushy—is one of the primary reasons that people do not find them flavorful or enjoyable. One way to identify that the *World's Healthiest Vegetables* are becoming overcooked is by their change in color. The *World's Healthiest Vegetables* start off with a bright beautiful color that can be enhanced after the first minute of cooking. But after about 5 minutes you will begin to see colors begin to fade and change, a visible sign that they are beginning to lose not only nutrients but flavor. Using a timer and following my directions for cooking times will help you avoid overcooking the *World's Healthiest Vegetables*.

I came up with an entirely new way of cooking the *World's Healthiest Vegetables* to take them from mushy to irresistible. My preferred methods for cooking the *World's Healthiest Vegetables* are Healthy Sauté and Healthy Steaming. Unlike traditional sauté methods, Healthy Sauté uses vegetable or chicken broth or water in place of the oil, which saves you calories since 1 tablespoon of oil contains 120 calories! To bring out the best flavor of the *World's Healthiest Vegetables* I use Healthy Sauté to cook cabbage, cauliflower, mushrooms, bell peppers, zucchini, and asparagus. (For more on Healthy Sauté, see page 121.) I use Healthy Steaming for broccoli, green beans, kale, collard greens, and other vegetables that require more moisture to improve their texture and flavor.

Just a few minutes of cooking over the recommended cooking times can make the difference between great tasting *World's Healthiest Vegetables* and those that have become overcooked and are no longer enjoyable. That's the reason I find using at timer is so valuable when I cook the *World's Healthiest Vegetables*.

Increasing Vegetable Intake

What I have found over the years is that people often have trouble trying to increase their vegetable intake because they just don't know how to make them taste good. I need to emphasize that it is not the vegetables themselves that don't taste good, but rather it's the result of how we cook them. I believe people enjoy vegetables made into cole slaw and salads because the vegetables are crisp and fresh. Cooked vegetables can have the same great flavor and similar texture if they are not overcooked. That's why I have spent many years creating ways to help you make cooked vegetables taste so good you will be asking for seconds and thirds. With my new cooking methods and recipes you will not be eating a plate of vegetables just because they are good for you or just because they will help you lose weight. You will be eating them because you love them. And the methods and recipes are also quick and easy that they will readily fit into your busy lifestyle (see page 124).

Tips to Make the World's Healthiest Vegetables Taste Great

Combined with cooking the *World's Healthiest Vegetables* at low temperatures for short periods of time, my new cooking methods also include the addition of one or two optional ingredients for extra flavor and nutrition. What's great about using these optional ingredients is not only do they make *World's Healthiest Vegetables* dishes more interesting but they also allow you to customize your recipes to meet your personal taste preferences. For example, if you want to enjoy a taste of Greece, broccoli with 1 TBS feta cheese and/or kalamata olives fits the bill and if you're looking for a rich Indian flavor, adding a little turmeric to your cauliflower may do the trick. Asian flavors have become increasingly popular, so some of my favorite additions to cabbage are ginger, a few drops of tamari (soy sauce), and/or rice vinegar. And friends have told me that our easy-to-prepare honey-mustard sauce has made Brussels sprouts a family favorite.

Cooking at Home Can Help You Save Money and Help Optimize Your Health

The current economic environment is affecting many of us these

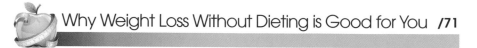

days. Did you know that cooking at home can be a great way to help save money and also help optimize your health?

Restaurant and fast foods are often nutritionally poor and not a bargain when you consider the lack of nutritional value you get for your money. Inflated portions and processed foods high in calories, fat, sugar, and sodium and low in vitamins, minerals, and phytonutrients are common fare when you eat out. It's no wonder that when you regularly make these foods the primary way to satisfy your hunger, you can end up gaining weight.

My new cooking methods will help inspire you to cook more of your meals at home because they not only taste great, but because cooking at home can also save you money. When you cook at home you know the quality of ingredients that went into your food, the calorie content, and that it was healthfully prepared.

When it comes to cooking the *World's Healthiest Vegetables* did you know they can lose from 50-80% of their nutrients when you use traditional ways of cooking? And they lose flavor as well! My recipes introduce you to my innovative cooking methods that not only retain the *World's Healthiest Vegetables'* maximum number of vitamins, minerals, and antioxidants,and also their vibrant color (a reflection of their nutritional content) but, best of all, they make the *World's Healthiest Vegetables* taste so great you will want to eat more of them! Even if you are not used to cooked vegetables being a little crisp, I think you will begin to love their texture and the extra flavor that comes with it.

Enjoy Foods that Help You Feel Full

You can eat as many the *World's Healthiest Vegetables* as you like —with no limit—and these vegetables can help you will feel full. You can eat them any time of day you feel hungry. Think about a cup of broccoli, bell peppers, or cucumbers, for example. These foods are rich in fiber that helps to fill you up and yet they contain minimal calories. One cup of broccoli has 31 calories, bell peppers 29, cauliflower 27, romaine lettuce 8, and cucumber 16. Eating plenty of low-calorie *World's Healthiest Vegetables* is a great way to help you curb your appetite.

Following Recipes Is Also Important

Of course, while keeping our calories to a minimum is important we need the experience of eating to be enjoyable as well. Unless the experience is enjoyable, we won't be completely satisfied. This is precisely why I have created the recipes to appeal to every aspect of the eating experience. In this book, I've provided you with over 50 recipes that look exquisite to the eye, taste delicious, and give you with the greatest nutritional value. The sheer pleasure of eating is high on my list of values! And most of my recipes take 7 minutes or less to prepare.

Calorie-Lowering Plan

I have found that one of the most difficult aspects about changing to a lifestyle of healthier eating is that people don't know where to begin. It all seems overwhelming at first. That's why I created the *Calorie-Lowering Plan* that combines the *World's Healthiest Foods* and my new way of cooking methods and integrates them into a menu of great-tasting recipes. People love these recipes because they take few ingredients, little time, and are easy to prepare. I have done all the work for you.

This Plan may help you prevent overeating by helping you to feel full. This means you may be less apt to feel hungry and crave those convenient, empty-calorie, often sugar- and fat-laden foods that usually work against weight loss.

For 4 weeks, you won't have to worry about what to eat for breakfast or what you'll cook for dinner. Everything is spelled out. I will

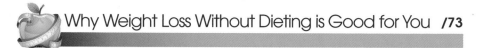

help you fill your plate with the *World's Healthiest Vegetables* that taste so great it will be easy to make them the centerpiece of your meals. And by the end of the 4 weeks you will hopefully have a really good idea of how to fit your personal tastes to a healthy eating lifestyle.

The Plan Provides 100% of Some Nutrients

The power behind the *Calorie-Lowering Plan* is its combination of nutrient-rich food, great taste, and ease of preparation. Nutrient-rich *World's Healthiest Foods* provide you with the many nutrients necessary to work synergistically and promote optimal health combined with taking in a minimum number of calories. And my health-promoting recipes help you to make delicious food in a matter of minutes. The Plan provides 100% of the following nutrients:

| over 100% for protein |
| over 100% for fiber |
| over 100% for vitamin A |
| over 100% for vitamin B1 |
| over 100% for vitamin B2 |
| over 100% for vitamin B3 |
| over 100% for vitamin B6 |
| over 100% for vitamin B12 |
| over 100% for vitamin C |
| over 100% for vitamin K |
| over 100% for calcium |
| over 100% for copper |
| over 100% for iron |
| over 100% for magnesium |
| over 100% for manganese |
| over 100% pantothenic acid |
| over 100% for potassium |
| over 100% for selenium |
| over 100% Zinc |

Enjoy Your Meals

Another important aspect of satisfying your appetite is to eat slowly and enjoy your meals. Take time for your meals and make them a celebration. If you focus on the foods you are eating, rather than just eating something to satisfy your appetite, you may feel more fulfilled and less hungry. Also, chew your food well as this allows for enhanced digestion and better absorption of nutrients.

Make sure you are giving your body time to register the satisfying effects of your meal. It takes about 15–20 minutes after consumption of most meals for your body to fully register the impact of the meal in terms of satiety (quenching of appetite). Sometimes people will feel continuing hunger during this period of 15–20 minutes that convinces them more food is needed. But if they wait for 20–30 minutes, this hunger will sometimes naturally subside.

Can I rely on my taste buds to tell me what my body needs?

Yes, if you work at it, you can rely on your taste buds to tell you what your body does and doesn't need. For most of us, however, trusting our taste buds is something that we will have to learn how to do, not something we can do right away. Here's why:

Our Taste Buds Detect Four Basic Flavors

First, when it comes to our body chemistry, we don't have taste buds for avocado flavor, or olive oil flavor, or strawberry flavor. Our taste buds are designed to detect only four basic flavors: sweet, salty, sour, and bitter. (New research is suggesting that umami, the sensation of savoriness, may be the "fifth basic taste.") Because we don't have taste buds for specific food flavors, our taste buds can't tell us directly which foods we need and which ones we don't. In addition,

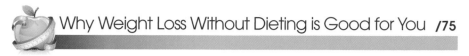

foods usually stimulate many of our different taste buds. Few foods only trigger our sweet taste buds, or our salty taste buds. Foods are usually complex in taste, and their impact on our taste buds is also complicated.

All Our Senses Enjoy Food

Second, the taste of a food is not determined exclusively from the reaction of our taste buds. The smell of a food, the visual appearance of a food, how we expect the food to taste, and how often we've eaten it previously all affect what we actually taste. When we sit down to enjoy a meal, it's not simply a question of our taste buds detecting four basic flavors. It's all our senses that enable us to enjoy our food, not just our taste buds.

Children Know Best

Some very interesting research studies of young, pre-school age children have tried to determine just how much our taste buds can be trusted. Children in these studies were selected because of their known, pre-existing vitamin deficiencies. For example, one study looked at children who were known to be low in vitamin D. These children were given a choice of several foods, but only one of the foods was high in vitamin D. For example, given a choice of orange juice (no vitamin D), soda pop (no vitamin D), and cod liver oil (high vitamin D), most of the kids actually chose cod liver oil! In other words, they seemed to be able to trust their taste buds. Many other studies, however, have repeatedly shown that even at a very early age, children tend to prefer the foods that their parents or brothers and sisters eat, and that the opinions of their family influence the way food tastes to them.

What Adults Should Do

How can we learn, as adults, to trust our taste buds? This task requires us to get back in touch with food. We have to give our taste buds a rest from all of the artificial flavors and artificial textures that are characteristic of processed food. We can't get back in touch with food unless we know what real food actually tastes like! The recipes in this book focus exclusively on real food. They are not only free from artificial flavors of any kind, but they are also created exclusively from whole, nutrient-rich foods. These foods will get you back in touch with real food and its taste. Careful handling and preparation of all foods is also emphasized in this book. The taste of real foods can be destroyed if the foods are not handled and prepared well. Getting back in touch with food means visiting the produce section of the grocery store more often and spending more time in our own kitchens.

Taste Buds: Reliable or Unreliable?

If you've had a hectic, stressful day where you didn't even get to sit down to lunch, and you stop at the gas station on the way home to get gas and see a bar of chocolate on the way out, you're in a very poor situation to trust your taste buds. In this kind of situation, your taste buds are going to tell you that a bar of chocolate is exactly what you need. But it isn't! What we all need is to respect ourselves and take the half hour lunch needed during our day to nourish our bodies with real food. But our taste buds can't tell us that. At the other end of the spectrum, if we've made most of our day's food selections form the World's Healthiest Foods, and we have taken time during the day to nourish ourselves with these foods, the opinion of our taste buds becomes much more reliable.

SECTION 2

Calorie-Lowering Plan

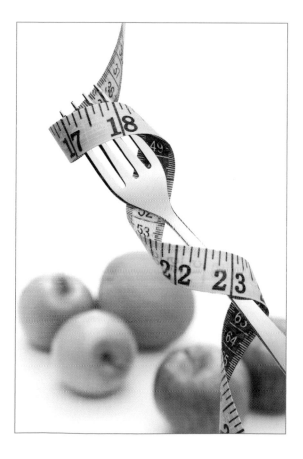

CHAPTER 6

Calorie-Lowering Plan

What to Expect When Following the Plan

In the U.S., adults consume an average of approximately 2,000 calories of food per day. On average, U.S. adults are also overweight,
and their intake of dietary calories is related to their overweight
status. Since my weight loss plan averages about 1,500 calories per
day, it represents a decrease of about 500 calories per day for the
average U.S. adult. Over one week's period of time—and all other
factors being equal—that 500-per-day calorie decrease would be
expected to result in a weight loss of about 1 pound. In one month, the
expected weight loss would be 4 pounds, and in one year, 48 pounds.

Regardless of the weight loss plan you follow, your daily calorie
intake must be matched up correctly with your activity level. If you
consume exactly the number of daily calories needed to complete
your daily activities (including exercise), you can expect to maintain
your current weight. If you exceed that number, you can expect
to gain weight. If you consume fewer calories than are needed to
complete your daily activities (including exercise), you can expect
to lose weight. Of course, in practice, weight loss never occurs with
this degree of mathematical exactness!

The amount of calories that a person expends by doing an exercise
depends upon personal factors such as their body weight. There
are numerous calorie expenditure calculators available on the
Internet,which you can use to figure out how much you will burn
by participating in different forms of exercise and activities.

Remember, before you embark on any exercise program, you'll want to check in with your physician who should be familiar enough with your health to give you personalized guidelines and any important do's/don'ts.

When following the Plan, you should expect to start developing a sense of foods, food groups, food selection, recipes, and menu planning that can serve as a springboard for development of your own ongoing weight loss approach that takes advantage of nutrient-rich, whole natural foods and that fits with your individual health status and lifestyle. You can also expect to get a sense of what a healthy, 1500-calorie diet feels like, and how it fits in with your other lifestyle goals. On a 1,500-calorie diet, many individuals will not be able to see weekly changes in their weight status unless daily exercise is incorporated into their weight loss plan.

How to Start the Plan

Welcome to the *Calorie-Lowering Plan*—a 28-day guide to help you lose weight. I believe that everyone can lead a healthy life and be slim, and that eating healthier affects how you feel, how much energy you have, and how healthy you are. I have created a complete Plan to help you lose weight, gain more control of your health, supercharge your immune system, and help rejuvenate your entire body. In this Plan you will discover some of the most nutritious foods around—The *World's Healthiest Foods*.

While you will likely feel the benefits during the first few days, know that it takes about 4 weeks for a habit to settle in. So give yourself this time and be patient with yourself as you embark on this *Calorie-Lowering Plan*.

Healthiest Way of Eating Journey

The Plan is not a diet nor an expensive, time-consuming program. It is a way to begin a lifestyle change to the Healthiest Way of Eating.

And I've done all the work for you so it's easy! I provide you with recipes that not only taste great but take only minutes to prepare— most take 7 minutes or less and you can make an entire meal in just 15 minutes! You just have to do the shopping and you don't have to break the bank to buy the foods called for in these recipes.

Before Starting the Plan

My 4-week, 1,500 calorie per day meal Plan will provide you with outstanding nourishment that is only possible with the nutrient rich-ness of whole, natural foods. The nutrient richness of your meal plan also draws upon its abundance of vegetables. Vegetables are your ticket to maximal nourishment for minimal calories. Even with the fantastic nutritional foundation provided by this meal Plan, you should not start the plan without observing the following guidelines:

- If you want to be certain that the diet Plan will meet your in-dividual nutrient needs, you'll want to consult with a registered dietitian or healthcare professional who has training and expe-rience in nutritional assessment. He or she will help you per-sonalize the plan to meet your unique personal needs. Because the Plan does not provide 100% of the Daily Value for all nutri-ents, it's also important to consult with a healthcare professional if you have any question about individual nutrient requirements brought about by your personal health status and/or health history.

- If you have kidney problems, it's important for you to talk with a physician before starting the plan. Even though it's limited to 1,500 calories of food, the Plan provides you with a generous amount of protein (mostly plant protein). While I believe that most people will benefit from this protein richness, the average daily protein level in this Plan (90 grams) needs to be evaluated by a physician for use by anyone with kidney problems. (Kidney problems often require implementation of a protein-restricted meal plan.)

- Depending on your current body weight and level of physical activity, a 1,500-calorie meal plan may not be appropriate for you to follow. If you have any question about this calorie level being a good fit for your level of physical activity or current body weight, you'll want to consult with a licensed healthcare professional before starting the plan.

Additionally, all of the following individuals need to consult with their healthcare provider before implementing our weight loss plan:

- All pregnant women, women who are nursing, and women who are considering becoming pregnant

- All individuals under 18 years of age

- All individuals who are concerned about obtaining Daily Value levels of nutrient intake for all nutrients based on diet alone and without the help of dietary supplements

- All individuals with special concerns about their intake of vitamin D

The Benefits of the Calorie-Lowering Plan

The Plan consists of 28 days' worth of daily menus that embrace the Healthiest Way of Eating. Since each of the breakfasts, lunches, dinners, and snacks for the week have a similar level of calories and nutrients, the Plan features a flexible approach that allows you to swap meals from one day to the next, if you would like. This will allow you to make the Plan work for your individual needs.

Healthier Lifestyle Tea

The Plan features Healthier Lifestyle Tea, which you drink before each meal. This tea is made from green tea and lemon juice. Green tea is not only delicious but is renowned for its health-promoting properties. These have been linked to a high concentration of catechin phytonutrients, which have a wide variety of protective benefits, many related to their potent ability to cleanse free radicals. Adding 1/4 teaspoon lemon juice per cup of green tea not only gives it a refreshing taste but additional benefits.

High-Energy Breakfast

Breakfasts feature good carbohydrates—primarily from fruits and whole grains—and delicious foods rich in protein—primarily from nuts, seeds, and eggs—to provide you with the energy you need to make it through the morning feeling satisfied, curbing your appetite until lunch. They offer you a supply of omega-3 fatty acids from walnuts and flaxseeds. Their appetite-satisfying qualities also come from the concentrations of dietary fiber that they provide.

Energizing Snack

Each day you'll enjoy energizing snacks that provide you with delicious tastes. Sweet fruits can help curb a sweet tooth and provide you with vitamins, minerals, phytonutrients and other nutrients while yogurt can provide extra calcium and protein.

Power Lunch

The Plan's lunches are delicious while keeping your appetite satisfied. They are a good mixture of protein, carbohydrates and good fats.

Most lunches feature a delicious salad, a great facet of a healthy weight loss approach. For example, one study found that women who ate a large low-calorie salad ate 12% less pasta even when they were offered as much as they wanted. Not only will your appetite be more satisfied but you'll also greatly benefit from all of the important nutrients it has to offer. Studies have shown that people who ate one large salad a day with dressing also had high levels of vitamin C and E, folic acid, lycopene and other carotenoids than those who did not add salad as part of their daily menu. All this without having to consume that many calories; for example, you could have as a base of a salad, 2 cups of romaine lettuce. This salad green features great taste and satisfying crunch, let alone a multitude of vitamins, minerals, phytonutrients, antioxidants and fiber. And it only contains 16 calories. Eating salads will curb your appetite allowing you to consume less calories over an entire meal.

In some of the lunches, you'll also find legumes and beans highlighted. These foods are so slow to digest that many people find them to be natural appetite suppressants. With their low glycemic index (GI) they keep blood sugar on an even keel and stave off hunger.

Good fats—like omega-3s from seafood and monounsaturated fats from extra virgin olive oil—are important to health on many levels including helping with the absorption of fat-soluble nutrients and phytonutrients. As a concentrated source of monounsaturated fats, you'll find extra virgin olive oil, which has antioxidant nutrients and also helps enhance the flavor of the dishes to which you apply it. Some studies have found that extra virgin olive oil can lead to small, but significant, loss of both body weight and mass.

Salad Dressing

While you may stock up on salad greens to further your weight loss-plan, the dressing you use may defeat all of your good intentions. Bottled dressing may not be only high in calories but contain excess sugar, salt, and preservatives. My solution is to use my Mediterranean dressing, which consists of extra virgin olive oil, lemon juice, salt, and pepper (and a little garlic, if desired, added in for taste and extra nutrition). My Mediterranean dressing will add great flavor to salads and will also enhance the taste of cooked vegetables—and contains all natural ingredients. Using small amounts of oil in your dressing may help you assimilate fat-soluble vitamins A, D, E, and K as well as carotenoid phytonutrients.

Let me say, though, that even though it may be more healthful than traditional dressings, you will still need to be very careful about the amount of Mediterranean dressing that you use. Olive oil (and other plant oils) has the highest calorie of all foods. It contains 240 calories and 28 grams of fat per ounce. When you make your Mediterranean dressing, be sure that you drizzle it very lightly on your vegetables and vegetable salads. A bottle with a very narrow-necked spout can be very helpful—especially if it lets you drizzle out only one or two drops at a time. If you do not control the amount of the dressing you use, you may end up adding too many calories to your daily intake.

Appetizers

One of my personal secret weapons to prevent overeating and, at the same time including more vegetables into my diet, is to start my lunch and evening meal with an appetizer of fresh vegetables such as cucumbers, carrots, celery, cauliflower, or zucchini.

Before the entrée, each dinner features an *Appetizer Satisfier* of crudité vegetables. This helps to curb your appetite before dinner (or lunch) so you are not starving when the entre arrives. One secret I discovered is to start enjoying the appetizers while I'm preparing the rest of the meal.

One of my favorite quick-and-easy *Appetizer Satisfiers* is prepared by tearing off a 4-5 leaves from a head of romaine. (When using the outer big leaves or romaine, I cut off the tips because they can be bitter and dry). Romaine hearts (romaine lettuce without the outer leaves), have a fresher and sweeter flavor than lettuce. Wash them, shake off the water, and sprinkle them with salt or dip them in salsa. And enjoy! Ancient Romans were known for eating this salted lettuce; in fact, our word for salad is derived from their name for this salted lettuce *salata*.

Slimming Dinner

Dinner is rich in fiber, which helps to curb the appetite as well as enhance digestion. You'll notice the inclusion of many herbs and spices—like ginger, cayenne, turmeric, mustard, and garlic—in the dinner recipes. Not only do they lend great flavor but they are rich in unique nutrients including those that help to promote beneficial digestion. As the dinners are satisfying yet not too heavy, they may also help you with a better night's sleep.

Almost all dinners include a *Green Power Side Dish*. These easy-to-prepare dishes consist of green vegetables that are at the cornerstone of changing to a healthier way of eating. These vegetables are so rich in chlorophyll and contain so many nutrients (including flavonoid and carotenoid antioxidants) but yet they have so few calories that they are essential to healthy weight loss. These nutrients will help support optimal metabolism because they provide your body systems with the nutrients it needs; if you don't have enough nutrients to support your metabolism, you won't be able to optimize your weight loss.

To give you an example of how important *Green Power Side Dishes* can be to healthy weight loss just think that if you ate two cups of green vegetables in place of a baked potato with butter or margarine, you would save over 300 calories! And since these foods are also low in GI they help balance blood sugar.

Sweet Desserts

Desserts are optional in the Plan, however, if you want dessert, I think fresh fruit is a great choice. They can satisfy a sweet tooth while, at the same time, provide you with a storehouse of health-promoting nutrients such antioxidants that help quench free radicals in the body. Choosing a healthy sweet dessert can really make a difference when it comes to weight loss; for example, a parfait made with low-fat yogurt and berries will save you 200 calories compared with eating one cup of ice cream.

Calorie-Lowering Plan

WEEK 1

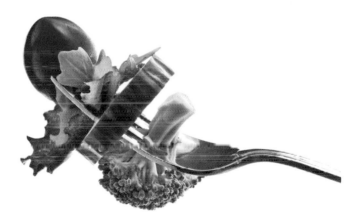

Week 1-Day 1

This day of the *Calorie-Lowering Plan* features easy-to-prepare menus, which offer exciting flavors and good nutrition; you'll enjoy plenty of delicious foods that will keep you satisfied. For the *High-Energy Breakfast*, you'll enjoy high-fiber cereal with fruit and nuts, for the *Power Lunch* a Mediterranean Caesar Salad, and for the *Slimming Dinner* tasty Salmon with Dill Sauce over Spinach. Along with these, you'll also enjoy *High-Energy Snacks* of an apple and orange; an *Appetizer Satisfier* of fresh crudites; a *Green Power Side Dish* featuring broccoli; and Healthier Lifestyle Tea. These meals are composed of nutrient-rich foods that give you many of the health-promoting nutrients you need every day.

Healthier Lifestyle Tea (pg. 126)
High-Energy Breakfast:
1 cup high-fiber cereal
½ cup blueberries
2 TBS chopped walnuts
1 banana, sliced
1 cup nonfat skim milk

Energizing Snack:
1 medium-sized apple

Healthier Lifestyle Tea (pg. 126)
Power Lunch:
Mediterranean Caesar Salad (pg. 137)

Energizing Snack:
1 medium-sized orange

Healthier Lifestyle Tea (pg. 126)
Slimming Dinner:
Appetizer Satisfier:
   1 cup carrot strips/slices
   1 cup celery sticks
   1 cup sliced cucumber
Salmon with Dill Sauce (pg. 154) served over 1 Minute Spinach 3 (pg. 161)
Green Power Side Dish
   5-Minute Broccoli 1 (pg. 165)

Week 1-Day 2

This day of the *Calorie-Lowering Plan* features easy-to-prepare menus, which offer exciting flavors and good nutrition; you'll enjoy plenty of delicious foods that will keep you satisfied. For the *High-Energy Breakfast*, you'll enjoy High Energy Breakfast Shake, for the *Power Lunch* Mediterranean Garbanzo Bean Salad, and for the *Slimming Dinner* Seared Asian Tuna. Along with these, you'll also enjoy *High-Energy Snacks* of an apple and yogurt; an *Appetizer Satisfier* of bell peppers, zucchini, and cauliflower florets; a *Power Side Dish* featuring red cabbage and Healthier Lifestyle Tea. These meals are composed of nutrient-rich foods that give you many of the health-promoting nutrients you need every day.

Healthier Lifestyle Tea (pg. 126)
High-Energy Breakfast:
High Energy Breakfast Shake
1 slice 100% whole wheat toast
½ cantaloupe

Energizing Snack:
1 medium-size apple

Healthier Lifestyle Tea (pg. 126)
Power Lunch:
Mediterranean Garbanzo Bean Salad (pg. 138)

Energizing Snack:
4 oz low-fat yogurt

Healthier Lifestyle Tea (pg. 126)
Slimming Dinner:

Appetizer Satisfier:
    ½ cup sliced red bell peppers
    1 cup zucchini slices
    ¼ cup cauliflower florets
    3 leaves romaine lettuce

Seared Asian Tuna (pg. 156)
Healthy Sautéed Crimini Mushrooms 1 (pg.175)
1 tsp sunflower seeds
Power Side Dish:
    Healthy Sautéed Red Cabbage (pg. 178)

Week 1–Day 3

This day of the *Calorie-Lowering Plan* features easy-to-prepare menus, which offer exciting flavors and good nutrition; you'll enjoy plenty of delicious foods that will keep you satisfied. For the *High-Energy Breakfast*, you'll enjoy a poached egg with Swiss chard, for the *Power Lunch* Romaine Salad with Goat Cheese and Mushrooms, and for the *Slimming Dinner* Spicy Asian Shrimp overmed Spinach. Along with these, you'll also enjoy *High-Energy Snacks* of papaya and pear; an *Appetizer Satisfier* of bell peppers, carrots, and cucumber; a *Green Power Side Dish* featuring broccoli; and Healthier Lifestyle Tea. These meals are composed of nutrient-rich foods that give you many of the health-promoting nutrients you need every day.

Healthier Lifestyle Tea (pg. 126)
High-Energy Breakfast:
3-minute Swiss Chard 2 (pg. 164) topped with 1 TBS pumpkin seeds and 2 TBS sunflower seeds and 1 poached egg, preferably omega-3-rich egg
1 slice 100% whole wheat toast
½ cantaloupe

Energizing Snack:
Papaya with Lime (pg. 128)

Healthier Lifestyle Tea (pg. 126)
Power Lunch:
Romaine Salad with Goat Cheese and Mushrooms (pg. 143)

Energizing Snack:
1 medium-size pear

Healthier Lifestyle Tea (pg. 126)
Slimming Dinner:
Appetizer Satisfier:
  ½ cup sliced red bell peppers
  ½ cup carrot slices/sticks
  ½ cup cucumber slices

Spicy Asian Shrimp (pg. 157) served over 1 Minute Spinach 3 (pg. 161)
Green Power Side Dish:
  5-Minute Broccoli 2 (pg. 166)

Week 1–Day 4

This day of the *Calorie-Lowering Plan* features easy-to-prepare menus, which offer exciting flavors and good nutrition; you'll enjoy plenty of delicious foods that will keep you satisfied. For the *High-Energy Breakfast*, you'll enjoy yogurt with fruit, for the *Power Lunch* Greek Salad with Garbanzo Beans and Feta Cheese, and for the *Slimming Dinner* Salmon with Ginger Mint Salsa. Along with these, you'll also enjoy *High-Energy Snacks* of orange and figs; an *Appetizer Satisfier* of celery, cucumbers, and carrots; a *Green Power Side Dish* featuring Swiss chard; and Healthier Lifestyle Tea. These meals are composed of nutrient-rich foods that give you many of the health-promoting nutrients you need every day.

Healthier Lifestyle Tea (pg. 126)
High-Energy Breakfast:
8 oz plain nonfat yogurt with 1 TBS blackstrap molasses
½ cup blueberries
½ fresh large papaya
1 medium banana
1 slice 100% whole wheat toast

Energizing Snack:
1 medium-size orange

Healthier Lifestyle Tea (pg. 126)
Power Lunch:
Greek Salad with Garbanzo Beans and Feta Cheese (pg. 133)

Energizing Snack:
2 dried figs

Healthier Lifestyle Tea (pg. 126)
Slimming Dinner:
Appetizer Satisfier:
> 1 cup celery sticks
> 1 cup cucumber slices
> 1 cup carrot slices/sticks
> 3 leaves romaine lettuce

Salmon with Ginger Mint Salsa (pg. 153) served over
Green Power Side Dish:
> 3-Minute Swiss Chard 2 (pg. 164)

Week 1-Day 5

This day of the *Calorie-Lowering Plan* features easy-to-prepare menus, which offer exciting flavors and good nutrition; you'll enjoy plenty of delicious foods that will keep you satisfied. For the *High-Energy Breakfast*, you'll enjoy a Tropical Energy Smoothie, for the *Power Lunch* a Mediterranean Turkey Salad with Mushrooms, and for the *Slimming Dinner* tasty Mediterranean Cod with Red Peppers and Basil. Along with these, you'll also enjoy *High-Energy Snacks* of a pear and grapes; an *Appetizer Satisfier* of zucchini, carrots, and cauliflower; a *Green Power Side Dish* featuring kale; and Healthier Lifestyle Tea. These meals are composed of nutrient-rich foods that give you many of the health-promoting nutrients you need every day.

Healthier Lifestyle Tea (pg. 126)
High-Energy Breakfast:
Tropical Energy Smoothie (pg. 130)

Energizing Snack:
1 medium-sized pear

Healthier Lifestyle Tea (pg. 126)
Power Lunch:
Mediterranean Turkey Salad with Mushrooms (pg. 140)

Energizing Snack:
1 cup red grapes

Healthier Lifestyle Tea (pg. 126)
Slimming Dinner:
Appetizer Satisfier:
>   1 cup zucchini slices
>   ½ cup sliced carrots
>   ½ cup cauliflower florets

Mediterranean Cod with Red Peppers and Basil (pg. 150)
Healthy Mashed Sweet Potatoes (pg. 174)
Green Power Side Dish:
>   5-Minute Italian Kale (pg. 171)

Week 1–Day 6

This day of the *Calorie-Lowering Plan* features easy-to-prepare menus, which offer exciting flavors and good nutrition; you'll enjoy plenty of delicious foods that will keep you satisfied. For the *High-Energy Breakfast* you'll enjoy high-fiber cereal with fruit, for the *Power Lunch* Chinese Chicken Cabbage Salad with Cilantro and Ginger, and for the *Slimming Dinner* Salmon with Mustard over the *Green Power Side Dish* featuring spinach; . Along with these, you'll also enjoy *High-Energy Snacks* of an orange and pear; an *Appetizer Satisfier* of cucumbers, bell peppers, and tomato served over and Healthier Lifestyle Tea. These meals are composed of nutrient-rich foods that give you many of the health-promoting nutrients you need every day.

Healthier Lifestyle Tea (pg. 126)
High-Energy Breakfast:

1 cup high-fiber cereal
¼ cup raisins
¼ cup strawberry slices
1 medium banana
1 cup nonfat milk

Energizing Snack:

1 medium-size orange

Healthier Lifestyle Tea (pg. 126)
Power Lunch:

Chinese Chicken Cabbage Salad with Cilantro and Ginger (pg. 131)

Energizing Snack:

1 medium-size pear

Healthier Lifestyle Tea (pg. 126)
Slimming Dinner:

Appetizer Satisfier:
      ½ cup sliced cucumbers
      ½ cup sliced red bell peppers
      1 medium tomato, sliced
      3 leaves romaine lettuce
Salmon with Mustard (pg. 155) served over
Green Power Side Dish:
      1-Minute Spinach 1 (pg. 159)

Week 1–Day 7

This day of the *Calorie-Lowering Plan* features easy-to-prepare menus, which offer exciting flavors and good nutrition; you'll enjoy plenty of delicious foods that will keep you satisfied. For the *High-Energy Breakfast* you'll enjoy Huevos Rancheros, for the *Power Lunch* Lentil Salad, and for the *Slimming Dinner* Chicken Breast with Rosemary, Thyme, and Sage. Along with these, you'll also enjoy *High-Energy Snacks* of an apple and pear; an *Appetizer Satisfier* of fresh crudites; a *Green Power Side Dish* featuring broccoli; and Healthier Lifestyle Tea. These meals are composed of nutrient-rich foods that give you many of the health-promoting nutrients you need every day.

Healthier Lifestyle Tea (pg. 126)
High-Energy Breakfast:
Huevos Rancheros (pg. 129)
½ large cantaloupe

Energizing Snack:
1 medium-size apple

Healthier Lifestyle Tea (pg. 126)
Power Lunch:
Mediterranean Lentil Salad (pg. 139)

Energizing Snack:
1 medium-size pear

Healthier Lifestyle Tea (pg. 126)
Slimming Dinner:
Appetizer Satisfier:
      ½ cup cucumber slices
      ½ cup fresh red bell pepper slices
      ½ cup fresh zucchini slices

Chicken Breast with Rosemary, Thyme, and Sage (pg. 148)
Healthy Sautéed Crimini Mushrooms 1 (pg. 175)
Green Power Side Dish:
      5-Minute Broccoli 2 (pg. 166)

Week 1 of the *Calorie-Lowering Plan* provides you with 100% or more of the Daily Value for 22 health-promoting nutrients and their health benefits for maintaining good health. The Plan will help you avoid nutrient deficiencies because, as you can see, it is built around nutrient-rich foods—rich in vitamins, minerals, hard-to-find omega-3 fatty acids, protein, fiber, antioxidants, and many other nutrients. The nutrient-rich foods in the Plan can provide nutrients in forms that are more available to you than most nutritional capsules. It is also an anti-inflammatory and immunity plan because it helps protect against inflammation, reduces free radicals, and bolsters the immune system.

Nutrients provided by the foods in the Plan perform many health functions in your body:

over 100% for protein	helps maintain healthy skin, hair, and muscles
over 100% for fiber	helps support intestinal regularity
over 100% for vitamin A	helps promote vision health
over 100% for vitamin B1	helps maintain energy supplies
over 100% for vitamin B2	helps protect cells from oxygen damage
over 100% for vitamin B3	helps promote cholesterol level balance
over 100% for vitamin B6	helps support your nervous system
over 100% for vitamin B12	helps prevent anemia
over 100% for folate	helps support heart health
over 100% for vitamin C	helps protect against free radical damage
over 100% for vitamin K	helps blood to clot normally
over 100% for calcium	helps build strong bones
over 100% for copper	helps promote proper thyroid function
over 100% for iron	helps keep immune system healthy
over 100% for magnesium	helps relax nerves
over 100% for manganese	helps supports your nervous system
over 100% molybdenum	helps protect against inflammation
over 100% for pantothenic acid	helps turn carbs and fats into useable energy
over 100% for phosphorus	helps in energy production
over 100% for potassium	helps lower risk of high blood pressure over
over 100% for selenium	helps protect cells from free radical damage

over 100% zinc	helps balance blood sugar
4.3 g soluble fiber	helps lower cholesterol levels
57.7 IU vitamin D	promotes bone health
2.0 g omega-3s	helps reduce inflammation
0.7 g tryptophan	helps promote better sleep
25,471 mcg beta-carotene	antioxidant that helps protect cells from free radicals
lutein&zeaxanthin	helps support vision health
lycopene	antioxidant that helps protect cells from free radicals
anthocyanins	antioxidants that help protect cells from free radicals

Calories, carbohydrates, fats, saturated fats, cholesterol, and sodium are lower than 100% DVs, which is desirable for most individuals.

Analysis for the following nutrients are not readily available: biotin, chromium, and iodine (found in sea vegetables).

You can get vitamin D from the sun; 15 minutes in the middle of the day will provide you your DV for vitamin D. Or, you can add 3.5 oz of sockeye salmon, which provides 247% DV for vitamin D, or 3.5 oz of ahi tuna, which provides 101% DV to your menu for the day.

Since there are no Daily Values for tryptophan, omega-3 fatty acids, and antioxidant like beta-carotene, lutein/zeaxanthin, lycopene, and anthocyanins, % DVs are not provided in the chart above.

The U.S. Food and Drug Administration's "A Food Labeling Guide" (US FDA, Center for Food Safety and Applied Nutrition/Office of Nutrition, Labeling, and Dietary Supplements, April 2008) was used as a foundation for the Daily Values we use to evaluate the Healthiest Way of Eating Plan. When you see the phrase "100% DV," it means that you are getting 100% or more of the Daily Value (DV). For more, see page 238.

Calorie-Lowering Plan

WEEK 2

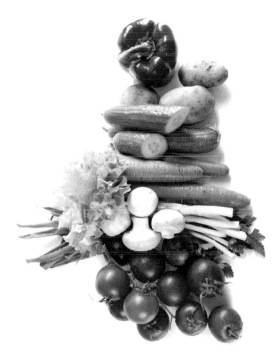

Week 2–Day 1

This day of the *Calorie-Lowering Plan* features easy-to-prepare menus, which offer exciting flavors and good nutrition; you'll enjoy plenty of delicious foods that will keep you satisfied. For the *High-Energy Breakfast*, you'll enjoy Poached Egg Over Spinach, for the *Power Lunch* Healthy Chef's Salad and for the *Slimming Dinner* Halibut with Ginger and Scallions. Along with these, you'll also enjoy *High-Energy Snacks* of an apple and orange; an *Appetizer Satisfier* of bell peppers, carrots and cucumbers; a *Green Power Side Dish* featuring Brussels sprouts, and Healthier Lifestyle Tea. These meals are composed of nutrient-rich foods that give you many of the health-promoting nutrients you need every day.

Healthier Lifestyle Tea (pg. 126)
High-Energy Breakfast:
Combine Healthy Sautéed Crimini Mushrooms 2 (pg. 176) with 1-Minute Spinach 1 (pg. 159). Top with 1 poached egg, preferably omega-rich egg
1 slice 100% whole wheat toast
½ medium cantaloupe

Energizing Snack:
1 medium-size apple

Healthier Lifestyle Tea (pg. 126)
Power Lunch:
Healthy Chef's Salad with Cheddar Cheese and Garbanzo Beans (pg. 134)

Energizing Snack:
1 medium apple

Healthier Lifestyle Tea (pg. 126)
Slimming Dinner:
Appetizer Satisfier:
      ½ cup sliced red bell peppers
      ½ cup carrot slices/strips
      ½ cucumber slices
Halibut with Ginger and Scallions (pg. 149)
Califlower with Turmeric (pg. 168)
Green Power Side Dish:
      5-Minute Brussels Sprouts with Mustard (pg. 167)

Week 2–Day 2

This day of the *Calorie-Lowering Plan* features easy-to-prepare menus, which offer exciting flavors and good nutrition; you'll enjoy plenty of delicious foods that will keep you satisfied. For the *High-Energy Breakfast*, you'll enjoy yogurt with fruit and sunflower seeds, for the *Power Lunch* a Healthy Waldorf Salad, and for the *Slimming Dinner* Healthy Sautéed Scallops. Along with these, you'll also enjoy *High-Energy Snacks* of an orange and figs; an *Appetizer Satisfier* of fresh crudites; a *Green Power Side Dish* featuring spinach and Mediterranean Medley; and Healthier Lifestyle Tea. These meals are composed of nutrient-rich foods that give you many of the health-promoting nutrients you need every day.

Healthier Lifestyle Tea (pg. 126)
High-Energy Breakfast:
8 oz plain nonfat yogurt
½ cup strawberries
3 TBS sunflower seeds
1 medium banana, sliced
1 slice 100% whole wheat toast

Energizing Snack:
1 medium-size orange

Healthier Lifestyle Tea (pg. 126)
Power Lunch:
Healthy Waldorf Salad (pg. 136)

Energizing Snack:
2 dried figs

Healthier Lifestyle Tea (pg. 126)
Slimming Dinner:
Appetizer Satisfier:
>   ¼ cup red bell peppers
>   1 cup carrot slices/strips
>   ¼ cup cucumber slices

Healthy Sautéed Scallops (pg. 145) served over 1-Minute Spinach 3 (pg 161).
Green Power Side Dish:
>   5-Minute Mediterranean Medley (pg. 172)

Week 2–Day 3

This day of the *Calorie-Lowering Plan* features easy-to-prepare menus, which offer exciting flavors and good nutrition; you'll enjoy plenty of delicious foods that will keep you satisfied. For the *High-Energy Breakfast*, you'll enjoy Poached Egg over Spinach and Mushrooms, for the *Power Lunch* Pineapple Chicken Salad, and for the *Slimming Dinner* Black Bean Chili. Along with these, you'll also enjoy *High-Energy Snacks* of yogurt and kiwifruit; an *Appetizer Satisfier* of carrots, zucchini, and cucumbers and Healthier Lifestyle Tea. These meals are composed of nutrient-rich foods that give you many of the health-promoting nutrients you need every day.

Healthier Lifestyle Tea (pg. 126)
High-Energy Breakfast:
Combine Healthy Sautéed Crimini Mushrooms 2 (pg. 176) with 1-Minute Spinach 1 (pg. 159)
Top spinach and mushroom with 2 TBS pumpkin seeds and 1 oz feta cheese and 1 poached egg, preferably -rich egg
1 slice 100% whole wheat toast

Energizing Snack:
4 oz plain non-fat yogurt

Healthier Lifestyle Tea (pg. 126)
Power Lunch:
Pineapple Chicken Salad (pg. 142)

Energizing Snack:
2 kiwifruit

Healthier Lifestyle Tea (pg. 126
Slimming Dinner:
Appetizer Satisfier:
      1 cup carrot slices/sticks
      1 cup zucchini slices
      ½ cup sliced cucumbers
Black Bean Chili (pg. 147)
¼ cup brown rice

Week 2–Day 4

This day of the *Calorie-Lowering Plan* features easy-to-prepare menus, which offer exciting flavors and good nutrition you'll enjoy plenty of delicious foods that will keep you satisfied. For the *High-Energy Breakfast*, you'll enjoy high-fiber cereal with berries and sunflower seeds, for the *Power Lunch* Mexican Cheese Salad, and for the *Slimming Dinner* 7-Minute Sautéed Chicken and Asparagus. Along with these, you'll also enjoy *High-Energy Snacks* of grapes and rye crackers; an *Appetizer Satisfier* of zucchini, bell peppers, and cucumbers; a *Green Power Side Dish* featuring collard greens; and Healthier Lifestyle Tea. These meals are composed of nutrient-rich foods that give you many of the health-promoting nutrients you need every day.

Healthier Lifestyle Tea (pg. 126)
High-Energy Breakfast:
1 cup high-fiber cereal
½ cup blueberries
¼ cup sunflower seeds
1 cup nonfat milk

Energizing Snack:
1 cup grapes

Healthier Lifestyle Tea (pg. 126)
Power Lunch:
Mexican Cheese Salad (pg. 141)

Energizing Snack.
2 rye crackers

Healthier Lifestyle Tea (pg. 126)
Slimming Dinner:
Appetizer Satisfier:
      1 cup sliced zucchini
      ½ cup sliced red bell peppers
      ½ cup sliced cucumbers
7-Minute Sautéed Chicken and Asparagus (pg. 146)
Green Power Side Dish
      5-Minute Collard Greens 1 (pg. 169) or Broccoli 1 (pg. 165)

Week 2–Day 5

This day of the *Calorie-Lowering Plan* features easy-to-prepare menus, which offer exciting flavors and good nutrition; you'll enjoy plenty of delicious foods that will keep you satisfied. For the *High-Energy Breakfast*, you'll enjoy Poached Egg over Mushrooms and Kale, for the *Power Lunch* Citrus Spinach Salad With Shrimp, and for the *Slimming Dinner* Halibut with Cauliflower and Fennel. Along with these, you'll also enjoy *High-Energy Snack*s of ½ a cantaloupe and yogurt; an *Appetizer Satisfier* of fresh crudites; a *Green Power Side Dish* featuring collard greens; and Healthier Lifestyle Tea. These meals are composed of nutrient-rich foods that give you many of the health-promoting nutrients you need every day.

Healthier Lifestyle Tea (pg. 126)
High-Energy Breakfast:
Combine Healthy Sautéed Crimini Mushrooms 1 (pg. 175) with 5-Minute Italian Kale (pg. 171) and top with 1 poached egg, preferably omega-rich egg
1 slice 100% whole wheat toast

Energizing Snack:
½ medium cantaloupe

Healthier Lifestyle Tea (pg. 126)
Power Lunch:
Citrus Spinach Salad With Shrimp (pg. 132)

Energizing Snack:
2 oz plain nonfat yogurt

Healthier Lifestyle Tea (pg. 126)
Slimming Dinner:
Appetizer Satisfier:
> ½ cup carrot slices/strips
> ½ cup cucumbers slices
> 1 cup zucchini slices
> 3 leaves romaine lettuce

Halibut with Cauliflower and Fennel (pg. 152)
Green Power Side Dish:
> 5-Minute Collard Greens 1 (pg. 169) or Broccoli 1 (pg. 165)

Optional Dessert: 10-Minute Berry Dessert with Yogurt and Chocolate (pg. 180)

Week 2–Day 6

This day of the *Calorie-Lowering Plan* features easy-to-prepare menus, which offer exciting flavors and good nutrition; you'll enjoy plenty of delicious foods that will keep you satisfied. For the *High-Energy Breakfast*, you'll enjoy Energizing Oatmeal, for the *Power Lunch* a Healthy Chef's Salad and for the *Slimming Dinner* tasty Miso Salmon over Swiss chard. Along with these, you'll also enjoy *High-Energy Snacks* of a kiwifruit and orange; an *Appetizer Satisfier* of bell peppers, zucchini, and cucumbers; a *Green Power Side Dish* featuring Brussels sprouts; and Healthier Lifestyle Tea. These meals are composed of nutrient-rich foods that give you many of the health-promoting nutrients you need every day.

Healthier Lifestyle Tea (pg. 126)
High-Energy Breakfast:
Energizing Oatmeal (pg. 124)
½ papaya

Energizing Snack:
2 kiwifruit

Healthier Lifestyle Tea (pg. 126)
Power Lunch:
Healthy Chef's Salad with Chicken, Cheddar Cheese, and Avocados (pg. 135)

Energizing Snack:
1 medium-size orange

Healthier Lifestyle Tea (pg. 126)
Slimming Dinner:
Appetizer Satisfier:
       ½ cup sliced red bell peppers
       ½ cup zucchini slices
       ½ cup cucumber slices
Miso Salmon (pg. 151) served over 3-Minute Swiss Chard 2 (pg. 164)
Green Power Side Dish:
       5-Minute Brussels Sprouts with Mustard (pg. 167)

Week 2–Day 7

This day of the *Calorie-Lowering Plan* features easy-to-prepare menus, which offer exciting flavors and good nutrition; you'll enjoy plenty of delicious foods that will keep you satisfied. For the *High-Energy Breakfast*, you'll enjoy Ground Turkey with Italian Kale, for the *Power Lunch* Tuna Salad Without Mayo, and for the *Slimming Dinner* Thai Scallops with Basil. Along with these, you'll also enjoy *High-Energy Snack*s of and apple and pear; an *Appetizer Satisfier* of zucchini and carrots, a *Green Power Side Dish* featuring collard greens; and Healthier Lifestyle Tea. These meals are composed of nutrient-rich foods that give you many of the health-promoting nutrients you need every day.

Healthier Lifestyle Tea (pg. 126)
High-Energy Breakfast:
Ground Turkey with Italian Kale (pg. 125)
1 slice 100% whole wheat toast

Energizing Snack:
1 medium-size apple

Healthier Lifestyle Tea (pg. 126)
Power Lunch:
Tuna Salad Without Mayo (pg. 144)

Energizing Snack:
1 medium-size pear

Healthier Lifestyle Tea (pg. 126)
Slimming Dinner:
Appetizer Satisfier:
      1 cup zucchini slices
      ½ cup carrot slices/sticks
      3 leaves romaine lettuce
Thai Scallops (or Shrimp) with Basil (pg. 158) served over the *Green Power Side Dish:*
      5-Minute Collard Greens 2 (pg. 170)
Optional Dessert:
5-Minute Ginger Pineapple (pg. 181) or 10-Minute Orange Treat (pg. 182)

Week 2 of the Healthy Weight Loss Eating Plan provides you with 100% or more of the Daily Value for 22 health-promoting nutrients and their health benefits for maintaining good health. The Plan will help you avoid nutrient deficiencies because, as you can see, it is built around nutrient-rich foods—rich in vitamins, minerals, hard-to-find protein, fiber, antioxidants, and many other nutrients. The nutrient-rich foods in the Plan can provide nutrients in forms that are more available to you than most nutritional capsules. It is also an anti-inflammatory and immunity plan because it helps protect against inflammation, reduces free radicals, and bolsters the immune system.

Nutrients provided by the foods in the Plan perform many health functions in your body:

over 100% for protein	helps maintain healthy skin, hair, and muscles
over 100% for fiber	helps support intestinal regularity
over 100% for vitamin A	helps promote vision health
over 100% for vitamin B1	helps maintain energy supplies
over 100% for vitamin B2	helps protect cells from oxygen damage
over 100% for vitamin B3	helps promote cholesterol level balance
over 100% for vitamin B6	helps support your nervous system
over 100% for vitamin B12	helps prevent anemia
over 100% for folate	helps support heart health
over 100% for vitamin C	helps protect against free radical damage
over 100% for vitamin K	helps blood to clot normally
over 100% for calcium	helps build strong bones
over 100% for copper	helps promote proper thyroid function
over 100% for iron	helps keep immune system healthy
over 100% for magnesium	helps relax nerves
over 100% for manganese	helps supports your nervous system
over 100% molybdenum	helps protect against inflammation
over 100% for pantothenic acid	helps turns carbs/fats into useable energy
over 100% for phosphorus	helps in energy production
over 100% for potassium	helps lower risk of high blood pressure
over 100% for selenium	helps protect cells from free radical damage
over 100% for zinc	helps balance blood sugar
9.7 g soluble fiber	helps lower cholesterol levels

29,680 mcg beta-carotene	antioxidant that helps protect cells from free radicals
400.5 IU vitamin D	promotes bone health
1.6 g Omega-3	helps to reduce inflammation
.84 g Trypothan	helps permotes better sleep
lutein&zeaxanthin	helps support vision health
lycopene	antioxidant that helps protect cells from free radicals
anthocyanins	antioxidants that help protect cells from free radicals

Calories, carbohydrates, fats, saturated fats, cholesterol, and sodium are lower than 100% DVs, which is desirable for most individuals.

Analysis for the following nutrients are not readily available: biotin, chromium, and iodine (found in sea vegetables).

You can get vitamin D from the sun; 15 minutes in the middle of the day will provide you your DV for vitamin D. Or, you can add 3.5 oz of sockeye salmon, which provides 247% DV for vitamin D, or 3.5 oz of ahi tuna, which provides 101% DV to your menu for the day.

Since there are no Daily Values for tryptophan and antioxidants like beta-carotene, lutein/zeaxanthin, lycopene, and anthocyanins, % DVs are not provided in the chart above.

The U.S. Food and Drug Administration's "A Food Labeling Guide" (US FDA, Center for Food Safety and Applied Nutrition/Office of Nutrition, Labeling, and Dietary Supplements, April 2008) was used as a foundation for the Daily Values we use to evaluate the Healthiest Way of Eating Plan. When you see the phrase "100% DV," it means that you are getting 100% or more of the Daily Value (DV). For more, see page 238.

Congratulations

Congratulations, now you have finished the first 14 days of the Plan. Like our Readers I believe you will start to see your body respond when you start eating more of the *World's Healthiest Foods* found in the Plan. You will also be feeling more alert and energized while starting to lose weight. Now that this way of eating has started to work, you should repeat the two weeks you have just finished to complete the 28-day *Calorie-Lowering Plan*. By the time you are done, you will be well on your way to a slimmer you. In Chapter 7 you will find practical tips for continuing your weight management.

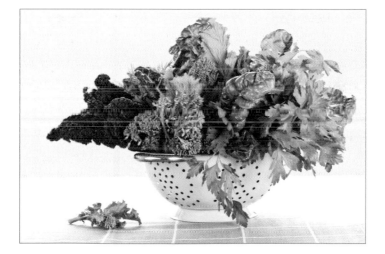

CHAPTER 7

Practical Tips for Continued Weight Management

Healthiest Way of Eating Tips for Weight Management:

Breakfast

Making time for a healthy breakfast sets the stage for healthy eating throughout the day. For most people, breakfast time comes at least 8-10 hours after their previous meal. So, in essence, while sleeping you have also been "fasting." In fact, the word itself, when broken down, means to "break a fast." When you wake up in the morning your blood sugar may be low or you may feel hungry. A general guideline is to have your breakfast contribute from 350 to 500 of your daily intake of calories.

It is important that breakfast fulfills some of your protein requirements for the day. You can do this by enjoying nuts, seeds, eggs, complex carbohydrates, and whole grain cereals as part of your first meal of the day.

When you select cereal it is best to look for one that is made from whole grains and has 5 grams of fiber per serving and not too much sugar or salt. Try not to eat foods that are high in refined carbohydrates (for example sugary cereals; pancakes, waffles, bagels, and muffins made from white flour; or white flour-based breakfast rolls or bars) first thing in the morning. These foods can cause a rapid spike in your blood sugar and may give you a short burst of energy but may cause you to "crash" an hour or two later.

What happens if you skip a healthy breakfast? If you don't give your body some real nourishment first thing in the morning, you may experience many unwanted consequences, including insufficient blood sugar levels and metabolic imbalances that leave you feeling sleepy or fatigued. And by the time lunch rolls around you will probably be so hungry that you will eat anything in sight! Several studies have found that skipping breakfast is a risk factor for becoming overweight or obese.

Many people say that they are not hungry first thing in the morning, which makes it difficult to eat breakfast. Eating a smaller meal for dinner will help increase your appetite for breakfast. If you don't have much of an appetite in the morning, begin the habit of eating breakfast by starting with something very small, such as a half a piece of whole grain toast with nut butter or a small bowl of whole grain cereal (with no added sugars!) with milk. As your body gets used to digesting food in the morning, you might notice a bigger appetite in the morning. Latest scientific studies show that those who eat breakfast everyday lost more weight.

Examples of a good breakfast:

Green Tea (Healthier Lifestyle Tea) with one of the following:

- Energizing oatmeal made with milk (or soy or rice milk) topped with blueberries and almonds
- Whole grain, breakfast cereal with fruit and nuts or seeds (sunflower or pumpkin)
- Poached eggs over spinach
- Healthy breakfast frittata

Healthiest Way of Eating Tips for Weight Management:

Lunch

What I have discovered as the answer to the dilemma of not having enough time to prepare a healthy lunch is to prepare a salad meal for lunch. Salad meals can provide you with all of the nutritional benefits of the Healthiest Way of Eating without having to cook! They take little time to prepare and the varieties you can enjoy are only limited by your imagination. To prepare a salad meal, you just need to assemble all of ingredients you want to include. These salad meals are not the "salads" that many of us grew up with consisting of a bowl of iceberg lettuce topped with tomatoes and French dressing. These are nutrient-rich, nourishing meals that can be prepared in just minutes using easy-to-find fresh ingredients.

I rediscovered the lost history of the classic Mediterranean-style salad while traveling the world to more than 80 countries, visiting people and cultures where there were traditionally few, if any, instances of the modern diseases that plague us today. These were countries where the people had come to expect the natural enjoyment of a long and vigorous life such as the Mediterranean countries, including the Greek Island of Crete. Salad meals were a large part of the diets in these areas. The Romans called them *salatas*.

Mediterranean-style salad meals are fresh, crisp, and delicious and there is absolutely no nutrient that cannot be obtained from them. It can be one of the most enjoyable meals of the day. In fact, a salad meal with a foundation of different types of lettuce and containing a wide variety of foods will often be closer to a "complete meal" than many other food possibilities. However, not all lettuce is created equal. The darker leaf lettuces provide you with more vitamins. And the lettuce in salads provides you with plenty of fiber so you feel satisfied and satiated. In addition, if you limit the amount of dressing, they can also be low in calories!

Here are some of your best salad green choices:

• Romaine lettuce	• Arugula
• Baby Spinach	• Watercress
• Green leafy lettuce	• Endive
• Red leaf lettuce	• Boston lettuce

Topping lettuce and salad greens with chicken, seeds, nuts, fish, shell-fish, or beans can provide you with more protein than a hamburger, twice as many nutrients as a traditional "entrée" plus two "side vegetables" as well as contributing hard-to-find omega-3 fatty acids to the salad meal. They can also be very low on the glycemic index.

Even small amounts of "garnish" type ingredients—like a table-spoon of pumpkin seeds or a sprinkling of walnuts instead of crou-tons—are a very worthwhile addition in terms of nutrients. Trace minerals and small amounts of high-quality omega-3 fats are nutri-ents that most U.S. adults don't get nearly enough of, and it doesn't take many pumpkin seeds or walnuts to bring some of these vital nutrients into the day's Healthiest Way of Eating.

Think of a salad meal as a canvas upon which you can mix the dif-ferent "colors" of foods. Depending upon your mood, the season, and the content of your refrigerator, you can make a salad with a mixture of your favorite lettuce. Starting with a nutrient-rich lettuce like romaine and adding a mesclun or spring mix variety of lettuces will create a great foundation for any salad. From there you can add in a selection of leafy greens, root vegetables, or other vegetables.

The sky's the limit as to what combination of nutrient-rich foods you can use. From there, you can add fruit, nuts, seeds, beans, legumes…the list of what you can add to a salad meal to make it delicious and nutritious goes on and on. Mix up a lot of different foods that feature a spectrum of nutrients and your salad bowl may provide you all the nutrients you need.

And don't forget the dressing. The reason is that the fats in dressings are necessary for our bodies to absorb carotenoids—the red, yellow, and orange pigments in fruits and vegetables, which act as antioxidants and prevent free radical damage that promotes aging and chronic disease. This is because carotenoids (along with vitamins A, D, and E) are fat-soluble, so our bodies cannot absorb them unless fat is present. Studies have shown that adding just a little fat to your salads can make a big difference in the amount of the protective compounds you absorb. people using full-fat dressing absorb twice the nutrients than those using reduced-fat dressing. And there was no absorption found among those using non-fat dressing!

Eating a salad meal is one of the most healthful eating habits you can adapt and one of the simplest. In just 5 minutes you can have a health-promoting meal rich in enough protein, healthy fats, vitamins, minerals, and powerful antioxidants to carry you through the entire afternoon.

Healthiest Way of Eating Tips for Weight Management:

Dinner

From a nutritional research perspective, there are three basic don'ts when it comes to dinner and how it might affect your sleep. First, don't make your dinner meal too large in size, especially when it comes to volume of food and amount of fat. It just takes too long for your stomach to empty large amounts of food. For example, some studies have shown that approximately 10-15 grams of fat in food can be processed in the stomach and passed on to the small intestine in one hour. It's not unusual for there to be 20 grams of fat in one fried chicken breast and another 30 grams of fat in one large serving of French fries. The 50 grams of fat found in those two foods alone might drag out digestion time in the stomach to 5 hours! If you ate these two foods for dinner at 8:00 pm, it might be 1:00 am before they even left your stomach. (During the nighttime, too much secretion of gastric acid in your stomach can be a factor that disrupts sleep.) As a general guideline, you'll usually want to keep your dinners in the 350-550 calorie range, and you'll want to keep your dinner food fats to about 10-15 grams. Typically, that will mean no fried foods and only a few tablespoons of fat-containing sauces and salad dressings.

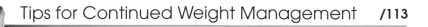

The second don't is related to the glycemic index. Although I've seen some research and some Internet discussion of high-glycemic index foods and their benefits for sleep, I believe that the best research here and the most healthful approach is to stick with low-glycemic index (low-GI) foods at dinner (and at other meals as well). Repeated studies have made it clear that low-GI foods at dinner can improve blood sugar reactions following breakfast the next morning and can help the entire next day start out in a way that is better for your blood sugar balance.

When you eat breakfast and lunch, your food needs to provide you with the nourishment and energy to get you through the rest of the day. When you eat dinner (unless you work a late shift, or have responsibilities that force you to change your schedule from the natural cycle of waking hours in the daylight and sleep hours in the dark), you are no longer trying to gear up for your day's activities. Instead, you are trying to prepare for a good night's sleep and wake up with a refreshed start to the next day. I believe that low-GI foods are the best way to help you accomplish this task. Green leafy vegetables, cruciferous vegetables, and salad-type vegetables (including lettuce, tomatoes, celery, bell peppers, radish, and cucumbers) have the lowest GI values of any food group and can be especially good choices here. On the don't list, however, would be processed and refined grain products (like breads and pastas not made from 100% whole grains) and sugar-added foods or drinks.

The third and final don't involves timing. You don't want to eat your dinner meal too close before bedtime. Your digestive tract works best when you are upright and sleep is not a good time for your stomach to be working in overdrive. If you keep your dinner meals in the 350-550 calorie and 10-15 grams of fat range I recommend, you should be able to eat your dinner meal approximately 3-4 hours before bedtime and have it work compatibly with your sleep.

As mentioned earlier, low-GI foods and moderate fat foods are good choices when it comes to dinner. In the low-GI category, you will want to focus on the type of vegetables described earlier: green leafy vegetables, cruciferous vegetables, and salad-type vegetables including lettuce, tomatoes, celery, bell peppers, radishes, and cucumbers. If you're going to include starchier vegetables like potatoes or green peas, I recommend keeping them to the 1 cup range in terms of serving size. Whole grains can also make good choices here, kept once again in the 1 cup range.

An important "do" when it comes to dinner is protein-containing foods. The combination of low-GI carbs and protein at a dinner meal has been shown in some research studies to help improve sleep, and there is some evidence that one particular amino acid—tryptophan— has a better chance to play a helpful role in our sleep-related nervous system activity when we combine dinner foods that provide protein and low-GI carbs. One very good protein choices here would be fish (but stay away from fried or breaded fish). If you enjoy and do well on lean meats, they can also be a healthy protein source and should be kept in the 4-6 ounce range at dinner.

Another "do" when it comes to dinner meals is the importance of a relaxed, enjoyable meal! Since dinner is coming at a time that is relatively close to bedtime, it's especially important to do thorough chewing of your dinner food and to relax in a way that will allow your body to engage in optimal digestion. This is one of the best time to savor the smells and textures and flavors of the *World's Healthiest Foods*.

Stick with some healthy protein choices (like non-fried fish) and low-GI (glycemic index) foods (like fresh green vegetables) at dinnertime. As a general guideline, keep your dinner meal in the 350-550 calorie and 10-15 grams-of-fat range. Don't go overboard on amounts for any food and leave a period of 3-4 hours between your dinner and your bedtime. And equally important, treat your dinner as the kind of meal that is designed to be especially relaxing and enjoyable.

Healthiest Way of Eating Tips for Weight Management:

Snacks

Healthy snacks contain an appropriate amount of protein, fats, fiber, and accompanying nutrients that will not only satiate your appetite so you will be less hungry between meals, but they also provide you with health-promoting nutrients to provide you with long-lasting energy.

Snacks should also provide energy and the feeling of satiety for the least number of calories. That's why I don't recommend popular snacks like energy bars because they contain excess amounts of fats and sweeteners, which contribute empty calories to your daily quota of calories. While a small amount of fat helps to maintain satiety, excessive amounts of fat can slow down your digestion to the point where it takes too long for you to derive energy and nourishment from your food. And excessive amounts of simple sugars can digest too quickly so you will be hungry in a very short time—much before the next meal. They also do not contain any fresh ingredients, which can help increase your energy and vitality.

An example of a healthy snack is fresh fruit (such as apples, pears, and blueberries) combined with nuts (such as almonds, walnuts and cashews) as it provides a good combination of fiber from the fruit and protein from the nuts (the latter increases the "holding power" of the snack). The fats from the almonds are a good addition to help slow digestive process and stretch the snack's impact. Fresh fruit and yogurt is also a great combination for a healthy snack. These snacks are not just good for you; they are less expensive than pre-packaged energy bars.

I'd like to add one last set of observations about individuals who find they snack too frequently. It's important to think about the pattern of your entire day in terms of enjoyment and activities. You may or may not want to make healthy snacking the solution to a daily pattern that just isn't working for you in terms of balance and enjoyment. In some cases, planning a larger, more nourishing meal before a difficult snack period time—and then shifting activities to turn a former snack period into a period of time focused on other enjoyable pursuits—can be a more effective way of "tiding yourself over" than experimenting with your snack content.

Healthiest Way of Eating Tips for Weight Management:

Appetizers

Even when I prepare dinner for myself I prepare appetizers such as broccoli and cauliflower florets, cucumbers, red bell peppers, zucchini, and leaves of romaine lettuce (romaine hearts) and serve them with a health-promoting dip such as tomato salsa. These are among the most healthy and easy appetizers to prepare. Extra virgin olive oil, balsamic vinegar, and low-fat yogurt also make great dips that require very little preparation. I enjoy these more than the more traditional soup and salad appetizer, and they can be more healthy and easier to prepare.

Even though it is not highly time-consuming to do the cutting and chopping of the vegetables yourself, you might want to consider the added convenience of pre-chopped and pre-sliced vegetables (although they are a bit more expensive). Many stores offer organically grown, pre-cut vegetables that could provide just the right amount of extra convenience to get you going on some improved appetizer options.

You will often find that it is often recommended to soak vegetables in ice water one hour before serving. I would avoid this practice as soaking leaches out many (about 20) of the nutrients found in the vegetables

Appetizers consisting of vegetables the take edge off of hunger and help you from overeating once the meal is served.

Healthiest Way of Eating Tips for Weight Management:

Beverages

Most people recognize, to varying extents of course, that what they eat (or don't eat) impacts their overall health. And, because of this recognition, many people try to eat more fruits and vegetables as well as less saturated fat and cholesterol while also cutting out junk foods.

However, it is important to remember that what you drink (or don't drink) also impacts your health. If you are careful to eat well, but drink excessive amounts of soda, fruit beverages, coffee, and/or alcoholic beverages you may not be as healthy as you could be. That is because such beverages contain a variety of substances that, when consumed in excess, are not health-giving. These substances include refined or artificial sweeteners, artificial flavorings, artificial colorings, synthetic preservatives, caffeine, and alcohol. In order to keep your beverage choices at the same peak nourishment level as your food choices, here are my recommendations:

Water: You can't go wrong with high-quality water. This beverage is not only at the top of my list, it is in a category all its own. While your water intake needs will vary from day to day, in its Dietary Reference Intake (DRI) recommendations, the National Academy of Sciences recommends about 13 cups of water each day for men and 9 cups for women. Space your intake throughout the day, make sure to rehydrate during and after exercise, and steer clear of excess water drinking during meal times if you find that practice to be personally helpful. For the highest quality water, I recommend attaching a high-quality filter to your tap water supply and drinking this filtered tap water as your primary source of water. To give yourself plenty of easy access to home-filtered waters, you may want to purchase an easy-to-carry water bottle and refill it whenever you are home so that you can have water with you when you are on the go. Look for glass or stainless steel ones. If you're getting a hard plastic (polycarbonate) bottle, be sure to purchase a "BPA-free" one. (BPA stands for bisphenol A, a problematic toxin that has often been added to polycarbonate plastics.)

100% Fruit Juices: Fruit juice can be healthy when it is 100% fruit juice, with no added sweeteners. But, keep in mind, that juice can pack a powerful punch in terms of calories and sugar, so it may not be wise to consume a lot of juice, even 100% fruit juice, if you are trying to lose weight or have blood sugar regulation concerns. To take full advantage of the nutrients available in the fruit, press or juice the fruit at home and consume it immediately. If you want to buy fruit juice at a grocery store, keep in mind that 100% fruit juice is harder to find than you might think as many fruit beverages sold in supermarkets contain only a small percentage (usually less than 10%) of actual fruit juice. For a special occasion, instead of serving soda, make a refreshing and healthy punch by combining sparkling water with 100% cranberry juice, ice, and orange slices with stevia (natural non-caloric sweetener) in a large bowl. (Remember though that while 100% fruit juice may be a healthful beverage, it shouldn't be thought of as a substitute for whole fresh fruit.)

Iced Herbal Tea: Instead of regular iced tea, treat yourself to a cool drink of herbal iced tea. Many herbs are rich in powerful antioxidants, which support the immune system and overall health. Brew the tea stronger than you would if you were planning to serve the tea hot and then add ice and a sprig of mint or a slice of lemon. Peppermint tea is wonderful when served cold. Or, try a combination of various herbs: chamomile, hibiscus flower, lemon grass, orange peel, rose hips, and strawberry leaf.

Healthier Lifestyle Tea: Healthier Lifestyle Tea is the name I have given to a delicious and health-supporting beverage made of one cup of green tea and one-quarter teaspoon of lemon juice. Green tea is not only delicious but is renowned for its health-promoting properties. These have been linked to its high concentration of catechin phytonutrients, which have a wide variety of protective benefits, many related to their potent ability to fight free radicals. Adding ¼ tsp lemon juice per cup of green tea not only gives it a refreshing taste but additional benefits. Lemon juice is a concentrated source of vitamin C, and hot water and lemon is a very cleansing and energizing beverage. If you are sensitive to caffeine, you can drink de-caffeinated green tea. Green tea is best enjoyed hot without sweeteners, however if you want to sweeten your green tea, stevia, agave nectar, or honey are your best choices.

Red wine: Red wine has been associated with health-promoting benefits. Always drink the wine with meals. Current recommendations are 1 glass for women and 2 glasses for men per day. If you cannot tolerate alcohol or choose not to include it in your diet, you can benefit from the resveratrol found in alcohol by enjoying alcohol-free red wine or purple grape juice.

CHAPTER 8

George's New Way of Cooking

From the time that I was five years old, cooking has been my passion. I studied at some of the greatest schools in the world including La Varenne in Paris, Guiliano Bugialli's cooking school in Florence, and Gourmet's Oxford in England. My experience cooking as well as in food development (when I ran Health Valley Foods) inspired my determination to create recipes and preparation techniques that enhanced the health benefits of foods. I call this style George's New Way of Cooking.

In addition to choosing the *World's Healthiest Foods* as mainstays of your Healthiest Way of Eating, it is important to cook them in ways that conserve their nutrient-richness. That's because the difference in nutritional quality between a food (let's say a vegetable, for example) that is cooked enough for it to have enhanced taste and texture compared to one that is overcooked and mushy is vastly different.

If you want to enjoy the full benefits that the *World's Healthiest Foods* offer, it's important to cook them for minimal amounts of time in order to preserve their health-promoting compounds. That's why you'll notice that most of the cooking recommendations for the vegetables in my book, *The World's Healthiest Foods: Essential Guide for the Healthiest Way of Eating* (and those I featured in the *Calorie-Lowering Plan*) entail only five or so minutes. In this short period of time you can cook vegetables *al dente*—tender on the outside, crisp on the inside—so that they have a delightful texture and vibrant flavor while maintaining so many more nutrients than if you cooked them for longer. Following my recommendations for the best cooking method and cooking time for each of the *World's Healthiest Foods*, as outlined in *The World's Healthiest Foods* book and the recipes included in this e-book, will ensure you'll enjoy great tasting foods that will provide you with great nutrition.

In addition to preserving nutrients during cooking it's important to cook foods using methods that don't create harmful compounds. For example, cooking with oil can oxidize their fats and cause lipid peroxidation products that can cause problems in the body and increase the risk of atherosclerosis. Instead of cooking with oil, I have come up with a healthy cooking method called Healthy Sauté that uses vegetable or chicken broth or water.

Healthy Sauté is a very special way of preparing foods because it has the benefits of three methods in one. It is a sauté that uses vegetable or chicken broth in place of heated oils; I am particularly conscious of creating recipes that do not use heated oils because they can potentially have negative effects on your health. It is like stir-fry because it brings out the robust flavor of foods but cooks them at a lower temperature. It is like steaming because there is enough moisture to soften the cellulose and hemicellulose, which aids digestibility. Healthy Sauté requires just a small amount of liquid to make the vegetables moist and tender. Vegetables such as cauliflower and asparagus, which only require a small amount of liquid to tenderize them, are especially good candidates for Healthy Sauté because steaming and boiling will dilute their flavor.

Healthy Sauté, Step-by-Step

- Heat 3-5 tablespoons broth or water in a stainless steel skillet.
- When broth begins to steam, add vegetables.
- Cover if necessary and sauté for recommended period of time.

In addition to reducing your exposure to oxidized oils, there is another great benefit of Healthy Sauté inherently important to healthy weight loss—the reduced consumption of calories. Just think typically you may use a few tablespoons of oil when you sauté vegetables. All you are really getting from the oil is the texture and oftentimes you don't really get much flavor. But two tablespoons of oil can add more than 200 calories to your meal. By using broth instead of oil to sauté, you can save yourself most of these calories. You probably don't disagree that that's a lot of calories that can be used in a better way.

One more note about oil: as you'll notice, extra virgin olive oil is a key component of the Mediterranean diet, and it is also one of the foods (and the only oil) included as a *World's Healthiest Food*. But I don't suggest cooking with it because its monounsaturated fats and polyphenol antioxidants can become damaged. Instead I suggest using it in salads and dressings, and drizzled on vegetables, fish, and chicken. (The highest heat I think it can take would be in the making of sauces.)

How to bring out the health benefits of alllium and cruciferous vegetables

After you cut your allium vegetables or cruciferous vegetables, if you let them sit for 5-10 minutes before cooking them you can help enhance their health-promoting properties.

Allium vegetables

The latest scientific research tells us that slicing, chopping, mincing or pressing allium vegetables (i.e, garlic, onions, and leeks) before cooking will enhance the health-promoting properties of garlic. A sulfur-based compound called alliin and an enzyme called *alliinase* are separated in the garlic's cell structure when it is whole. Cutting garlic ruptures the cells and releases these elements allowing them to come in contact and form a powerful new compound called allicin which not only adds to the number of garlic's health-promoting benefits but is also the culprit behind their pungent aroma and gives garlic its "bite."

When it comes to garlic, the more finely it is chopped, the more alliicin is produced. Pressing garlic or mincing them into a smooth paste will give you the strongest flavor and the greatest amount of alliicin. The stronger the smell and flavor of garlic, the more health-promoting nutrients it contains. So the next time you chop, mince or press your garlic, you may have a greater appreciation of its strong aroma knowing that the more pungent the smell the better it is for your health!

Because this process takes some time, I recommend letting garlic sit for about 5-10 minutes after cutting while you prepare other ingredients. This is to ensure the maximum synthesis of alliicin. Once the compounds are formed they are quite stable and will withstand low heat for a short period of time, approximately 15 minutes. Research on garlic reinforces the validity of this practice. When crushed garlic was heated its ability to inhibit cancer development in animals was blocked; yet, when the researchers allowed the crushed garlic to "stand" for 10 minutes before heating, its anti-cancer activity was preserved.

Cruciferous vegetables

Research also shows that cutting cruciferous vegetables (i.e., cabbage, kale, broccoli, cauliflower, Brussels sprouts, collard greens, etc.) into small pieces breaks down cell walls and enhances the activation of an enzyme called myrosinase that slowly converts some of the plant nutrients into their active forms, which have been shown to contain health-promoting properties. So, to get the enhanced benefits from these vegetables, let them sit for a minimum of 5 minutes, optimally 10 minutes, after cutting, before eating or cooking.

Cooking at low or medium heat for short periods of time (up to 15 minutes) should not destroy the active phytonutrients since once they are formed, they are fairly stable.

CHAPTER 9

Recipes
Breakfast and Snacks

Energizing Oatmeal

A perfect way to start the day! And who would have thought that a bowl of oatmeal could provide so many nutrients to your *Calorie-Lowering Plan.*

Ingredients:

1 cup water
½ cup old fashioned rolled oats
½ apple, chopped
2 TBS raisins
2 TBS dried cranberries
¼ tsp cinnamon
½ TBS ground flax seeds
½ TBS chopped walnuts
½ cup nonfat milk
½ TBS blackstrap molasses

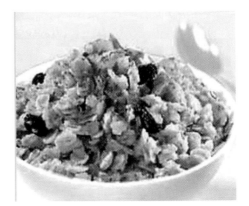

Directions:

1.   Bring the water and salt to a boil in a saucepan, then turn the heat to low and add the oats, chopped apple, raisins, and dried cranberries.

2.   Cook for about 5 minutes, stirring regularly so that the oatmeal will not clump together. Add cinnamon, flax seeds, and walnuts, stir, cover the pan and turn off heat. Let sit for 5 minutes. Serve with milk and molasses.

Serves 1

Nutritional Profile							
Calories	429	Carbohydrates	86.44 g	Saturated Fat	0.93 g	Calcium	208.03 mg
Calories-Saturated Fat	8	Dietary Fiber	9.47 g	Fat - Total	7.06 g	Potassium	650.64 mg
Protein	11.41 g	Soluble Fiber	2.17 g	Cholesterol	2.45 mg	Sodium	58.33 mg

Ground Turkey with Italian Kale

Include Italian kale for breakfast—
it's a great way to add nutrition to
your *Calorie-Lowering* menu.

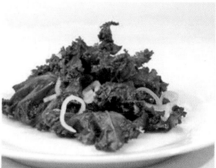

Ingredients:

1 clove garlic, chopped

¼ medium onion, chopped

2 TBS low-sodium chicken or
vegetable broth

2 oz-wt low-fat ground turkey

3 cups Italian kale (or any variety) sliced 1/8" thick

Sea salt and pepper to taste

Directions:

1. Chop garlic and onion and let sit for at least 5 minutes to bring out
    their health-promoting properties.

2. Heat 2 TBS broth on medium heat. Add onion and sauté for 3
    minutes, stirring frequently.

3. Add garlic and turkey and cook for an additional 3 minutes breaking
    up the clumps of turkey.

4. Steam kale for 5 minutes.

5. For best taste cut again into smaller pieces and combine with
    turkey mixture.

Serves 1

Nutritional Profile							
Calories	252	Carbohydrates	23.86 g	Saturated Fat	2.15 g	Calcium	297.88 mg
Calories-Saturated Fat	19	Dietary Fiber	4.55 g	Fat - Total	9.00 g	Potassium	1116.64 mg
Protein	22.94 g	Soluble Fiber	1.61 g	Cholesterol	57.83 mg	Sodium	153.21 mg

Healthier Lifestyle Tea

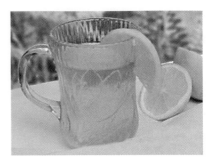

Healthier Lifestyle Tea is green tea with lemon. It's a very cleansing and energizing way to start the day. If you're sensitive to caffeine, you can drink decaffeinated green tea.

Green tea is not only delicious but is renowned for its health-promoting properties. These have been linked to its high concentration of catechin phytonutrients, which have a wide variety of protective benefits, many related to their potent ability to fight free radicals. Adding ¼ tsp lemon juice per cup of green tea not only gives it a refreshing taste but additional benefits. Lemon juice is a concentrated source of vitamin C, and hot water and lemon is a very cleansing and energizing beverage

Ingredients:

1 cup green tea
¼ tsp lemon juice

Directions:

1. Fill a non-reactive pot or pan (glass or stainless steel) with water and bring to "boil".
2. Measure 1 tsp of green tea into a sieve or tea ball and place in 1 cup hot water.
3. Let steep for 2-3 minutes and add lemon juice. Steeping too long will make it bitter.

Serves 1

Nutritional Profile							
Calories	0	Carbohydrates	0.11 g	Saturated Fat	0 g	Calcium	0.09 mg
Calories-Saturated Fat	0	Dietary Fiber	0.01 g	Fat - Total	0 g	Potassium	26.58 mg
Protein	0g	Soluble Fiber	0 g	Cholesterol	0 mg	Sodium	0.01 mg

High-Energy Breakfast Shake

Quick, easy, and healthy—
a great way to start the day

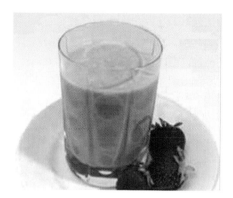

Ingredients:

1 TBS sunflower seeds
½ medium banana
¼ cup whole strawberries
1 cups nonfat milk
½ TBS almond butter
1 TBS ground flaxseeds
½ TBS blackstrap molasses
½ large papaya

Directions:

Grind sunflower seeds and add rest of ingredients and blend until smooth.

Serves 1

Nutritional Profile							
Calories	377	Carbohydrates	59.97 g	Saturated Fat	1.48 g	Calcium	420.66 mg
Calories-Saturated Fat	13	Dietary Fiber	8.63 g	Fat - Total	11.20 g	Potassium	1400.75 mg
Protein	11 g	Soluble Fiber	0.19 g	Cholesterol	0.00 mg	Sodium	151.35 mg

Papaya with Lime (or substitute grapefruit for papaya)

Rich in vitamin C, potassium, and folate, papayas are also low in calories making them a great addition to the *Calorie-Lowering Plan.*

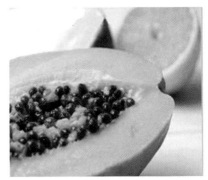

Ingredients:

½ medium papaya (or ½ grapefruit)
½ TBS lime juice
1/8 tsp lime zest

Directions:

Cut papaya in half and serve with lime juice and zest.

Serves 1

Nutritional Profile							
Calories	61	Carbohydrates	15.55 g	Saturated Fat	0.07 g	Calcium	37.54 mg
Calories-Saturated Fat	1	Dietary Fiber	2.77 g	Fat - Total	0.22 g	Potassium	399.49 mg
Protein	0.96 g	Soluble Fiber	NV	Cholesterol	0 mg	Sodium	4.71 mg

Poached Huevos Rancheros

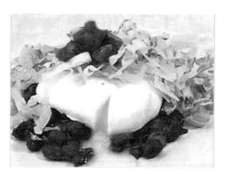

Add an international flavor to your breakfast menu with this easy-to-prepare version of a popular Mexican dish that will add both flavor and nutrition to your *Weight Loss Success* menu.

Ingredients:

1½ TBS low-sodium chicken or vegetable broth
1 cup cooked black beans (or half of 15 oz can of black beans, drained)
½ tsp ground cumin
1 tsp red chili powder
1 TBS chopped fresh cilantro
Salt and black pepper to taste
1 cup shredded romaine lettuce
¼ large avocado, cubed
1 TBS prepared salsa
Serve with 1 poached egg, preferably omega-rich eggs

Directions:

1.   Heat broth, beans, cumin, and red chili powder for about 10 minutes on medium low heat, stirring occasionally. Add cilantro, salt, and pepper.

2.   Serve beans with poached egg, salsa, shredded romaine lettuce, and avocado.

Serves 1

Nutritional Profile							
Calories	363	Carbohydrates	45.09 g	Saturated Fat	2.31 g	Calcium	179.48 mg
Calories-Saturated Fat	21	Dietary Fiber	15.60 g	Fat - Total	11.57 g	Potassium	994.03 mg
Protein	23.09 g	Soluble Fiber	0 g	Cholesterol	211 mg	Sodium	267.87 mg

Tropical Energy Smoothie

Add a bit of the tropics to your *Calorie-Lowering Plan* with this quick-and-easy smoothie; the tahini adds protein to help carry you through the morning.

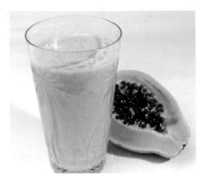

Ingredients:

1 TBS tahini
½ medium ripe banana
½ cup non-fat plain yogurt
3/4 cups pineapple juice
½ medium papaya

Directions:

Scoop out flesh from papaya with spoon and add to blender with rest of ingredients. Blend until smooth. .

Serves 1 (8 oz. glass)

Nutritional Profile							
Calories	377	Carbohydrates	64.37 g	Saturated Fat	2.48 g	Calcium	309.13 mg
Calories-Saturated Fat	22	Dietary Fiber	5.35 g	Fat - Total	10.48 g	Potassium	1201.11 mg
Protein	11.29 g	Soluble Fiber	0.11 g	Cholesterol	7.35 mg	Sodium	99.90 mg

Recipes
Lunch and Salads

Chinese Chicken Cabbage Salad

Like other members of the cabbage family Chinese cabbage is low in calories but boasts greater B vitamins, folate. It also contains incredible amounts of zinc.

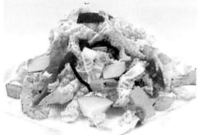

Photo shown with sea vegetable and red bell peppers

Ingredients:

4 cups Napa cabbage, sliced thin
½ tsp tamari (soy saucc)
½ TBS minced ginger
1 medium cloves garlic, pressed
¼ cup chopped cilantro
2 oz-wt cooked chicken breast, shredded or cut into 1" cubes
¼ medium avocado, sliced
1 TBS extra virgin olive oil
1 TBS rice vinegar
Salt and pepper to taste

Directions:

Combine all salad ingredients and then toss with olive and vincgar.

Serves 1

Nutritional Profile							
Calories	477	Carbohydrates	22.84 g	Saturated Fat	4.51 g	Calcium	282.86 mg
Calories-Saturated Fat	41	Dietary Fiber	7.17 g	Fat - Total	28.26 g	Potassium	502.09 mg
Protein	35.54 g	Soluble Fiber	0.03 g	Cholesterol	72.29 mg	Sodium	273.34 mg

Citrus Spinach Salad With Shrimp

Baby spinach has become a favorite salad ingredient. Enjoy this low calorie, nutritious salad; the orange will give you a big boost of vitamin C!

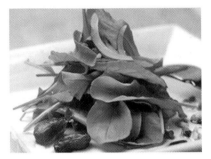

Photo shown without shrimp and orange wedges

Ingredients:

6 cups fresh baby spinach

1 medium orange, cut segments into small pieces

1 TBS chopped dates

3 oz-wt cooked shrimp

1 TBS slivered almonds

1 TBS lemon juice

1 TBS extra virgin olive oil

Salt and pepper to taste

Directions:

Combine all salad ingredients and toss with lemon juice and extra virgin olive oil.

Serves 1

Nutritional Profile							
Calories	423	Carbohydrates	43.49 g	Saturated Fat	2.29 g	Calcium	248.23 mg
Calories-Saturated Fat	21	Dietary Fiber	11.90 g	Fat - Total	19.07 g	Potassium	667.79 mg
Protein	28.00 g	Soluble Fiber	2.22 g	Cholesterol	172.12 mg	Sodium	475.73 mg

Greek Salad with Garbanzo Beans and Feta Cheese

Salads with garbanzo beans are among the favorites along the Mediterranean. This version is not only nutritious with great flavor, but the addition of the mint makes it wonderfully refreshing as well.

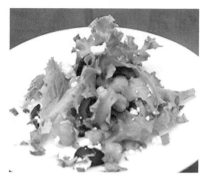

Ingredients:

6 cups mixed greens salad
½ cup fresh peppermint
1 oz reduced-fat feta cheese
¾ cup cooked garbanzo beans or
    canned (No-BPA), rinsed and drained
1 tsp sunflower seeds
¼ medium avocado
Salt and pepper to taste
1 TBS extra virgin olive oil
1 TBS red wine vinegar

Directions:

Combine all salad ingredients and then toss with olive oil and vinegar.

Serves 1

Nutritional Profile							
Calories	524	Carbohydrates	52.72 g	Saturated Fat	5.31 g	Calcium	305.16 mg
Calories-Saturated Fat	48	Dietary Fiber	9.93 g	Fat - Total	27.20 g	Potassium	2128.66 mg
Protein	25.05 g	Soluble Fiber	0 g	Cholesterol	8.34 mg	Sodium	452.31 mg

Healthy Chef's Salad with Cheddar Cheese and Garbanzo Beans

Variety is of key importance to enjoying and sticking to your *Calorie-Lowering* menu. This salad is a great example of how innovative you can become in creating a delicious salad that is low in calories.

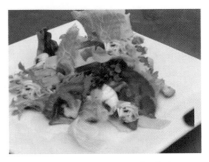

Not all ingredients shown in photo

Ingredients:

4 cups mixed greens salad
1 oz low-fat cheddar cheese, shredded
¼ cup sliced cucumber, unpeeled
¼ cup red ripe tomato
¼ cup fresh sweet red bell peppers, chopped
¼ cup avocado, diced
½ cup cooked garbanzo beans or
        canned (No-BPA), rinsed and drained
½ cup crimini mushrooms, sliced
¼ cup raisins
½ TBS extra virgin olive oil
½ TBS balsamic vinegar or lemon juice
Salt and pepper to taste

Directions:

Combine all salad ingredients and then toss with olive oil and vinegar or lemon juice.

Serves 1

Nutritional Profile							
Calories	439	Carbohydrates	56.14 g	Saturated Fat	3.30 g	Calcium	274.25 mg
Calories-Saturated Fat	30	Dietary Fiber	11.05 g	Fat - Total	17.85 g	Potassium	1987.87 mg
Protein	21.79 g	Soluble Fiber	2.05 g	Cholesterol	5.95 mg	Sodium	201.74 mg

Healthy Chef's Salad with Chicken, Cheddar Cheese and Avocados

I love salads. Delicious, nutritious, satisfying and refreshing! The protein provided by the chicken and cheddar cheese will help keep you satisfied until your mid-day snack.

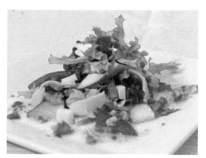

Not all ingredients shown in photo; walnuts added

Ingredients:

6 cups mixed greens salad
2 oz chicken breast, shredded or cubed
½ oz low-fat cheddar cheese, shredded
¼ cup sliced cucumbers
¼ cup tomatoes, diced
¼ cup red bell peppers diced
¼ cup fresh crimini mushrooms, sliced
¼ medium avocado, sliced
¼ cup frozen green peas, thawed
¼ cup cooked garbanzo beans or
        canned (No BPA), rinsed and drained
½ TBS extra virgin olive oil
½ TBS lemon juice
Salt and pepper to taste

Directions:

Combine all salad ingredients and then toss with olive oil and lemon juice.

Serves 1

Nutritional Profile							
Calories	437	Carbohydrates	39.71 g	Saturated Fat	2.87 g	Calcium	245 mg
Calories-Saturated Fat	26	Dietary Fiber	7.51 g	Fat - Total	17.84 g	Potassium	2354.31 mg
Protein	35.98 g	Soluble Fiber	0.31 g	Cholesterol	51.17 mg	Sodium	191.36 mg

Healthy Waldorf Salad

This low-calorie version of the classic Waldorf salad not only satisfies your hunger, but it is easy to prepare and tastes great!

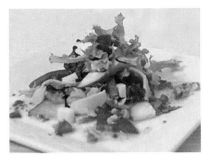

Not all ingredients shown; cucumbers and tomatoes added

Ingredients:

½ medium apple, chopped
½ stalk celery, diced
2 oz-wt chicken breast, diced
1 TBS walnuts, chopped
1 TBS sunflower seeds
1 TBS parsley, chopped
1 tsp extra virgin olive oil
1 TBS lemon juice
6 cups mixed salad greens
Salt and pepper to taste

Directions:

Combine all ingredients except for salad greens and then serve over the salad greens.

Serves 1

Nutritional Profile							
Calories	471	Carbohydrates	52.46 g	Saturated Fat	2.27 g	Calcium	212.80 mg
Calories-Saturated Fat	20	Dietary Fiber	10.34 g	Fat - Total	16.70 g	Potassium	2160.59 mg
Protein	34.59 g	Soluble Fiber	2.34 g	Cholesterol	48.19 mg	Sodium	93.22 mg

Mediterranean Caesar Salad

One of the benefits of the Mediterranean-style of eating is its abundance of vegetables and legumes, which provide rich sources of dietary fiber that help you feel satiated and satisfied—an important factor in any *Calorie-Lowering Plan.*

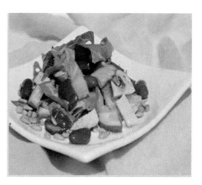

Ingredients:

6 cups romaine lettuce
1 medium red tomato, sliced or diced
¼ cup sliced cucumbers with peel
¾ cup cooked kidney beans or
        canned (No BPA), rinsed and drained
½ cup sliced crimini mushrooms
1 TBS grated Parmesan cheese
2 TBS sunflower seeds

Dressing:
2 TBS lemon juice
½ TBS extra virgin olive oil
1 garlic cloves, chopped (optional)
Salt and pepper to taste

Directions:

Combine all ingredients and toss with dressing ingredients. Dressing ingredients don't have to be combined separately before tossing.

Serves 1

Nutritional Profile							
Calories	403	Carbohydrates	50.92 g	Saturated Fat	3.03 g	Calcium	270.52 mg
Calories-Saturated Fat	27	Dietary Fiber	24.43 g	Fat - Total	15.10 g	Potassium	1903.65 mg
Protein	22.85 g	Soluble Fiber	0.07 g	Cholesterol	4.40 mg	Sodium	131.16 mg

Mediterranean Garbanzo Bean Salad

Legumes, such as garbanzo beans, provide a great combination of protein and fiber—both of which help you remain feeling satisfied until your next meal.

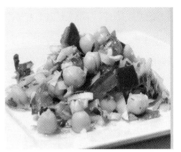

Ingredients:

6 cups salad greens
3/4 cup cooked garbanzo beans or
    canned (No BPA), rinsed and drained
2 TBS red onion, chopped
1 TBS Parmesan cheese
1 medium tomato, chopped
1 TBS extra virgin olive oil
1 TBS lemon juice
Salt and pepper to taste

Directions:

Combine all salad ingredients and toss with olive oil and lemon juice.

Serves 1

Nutritional Profile							
Calories	441	Carbohydrates	54.80 g	Saturated Fat	2.91 g	Calcium	277.15 mg
Calories-Saturated Fat	26	Dietary Fiber	9.38 g	Fat - Total	18.54 g	Potassium	2263.11 mg
Protein	20.50 g	Soluble Fiber	0.03 g	Cholesterol	4.40 mg	Sodium	141.99 mg

Mediterranean Lentil Salad

Unlike beans, lentils don't require soaking before cooking and can be prepared in 20-30 minutes. They provide you with a great source of molybdenum and folate in your *Calorie-Lowering Plan*.

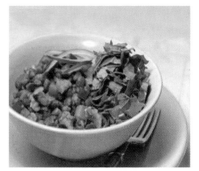

Ingredients:

1 cup cooked lentils
¼ medium red onion, chopped
1 clove garlic, chopped
¼ cup tomatoes, diced
¼ cup red bell pepper, diced
1 tsp fresh lemon juice
½ TBS extra virgin olive oil
2 TBS sunflower seeds
Salt and pepper to taste
2 cups romaine lettuce, chopped

Directions:

1. Chop garlic and let sit for 5 minutes to bring out its health-promoting properties.
2. Combine all ingredients (except romaine)and toss. Serve with romaine lettuce.

Serves 1

Nutritional Profile							
Calories	380	Carbohydrates	52.71 g	Saturated Fat	1.68 g	Calcium	95.36 mg
Calories-Saturated Fat	15	Dietary Fiber	20.21 g	Fat - Total	11.03 g	Potassium	1206.53 mg
Protein	21.79 g	Soluble Fiber	2.58 g	Cholesterol	0 mg	Sodium	16.88 mg

Mediterranean Turkey Salad with Mushrooms

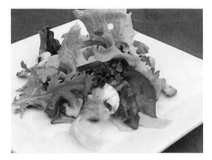

If you want to add more selenium, niacin, and copper to your *Calorie-Lowering Plan*, you may be surprised that crimini mushrooms are an excellent source of these important nutrients.

Ingredients:

6 cups salad greens
½ medium tomato, diced
½ cup sliced cucumbers
4 kalamata olives
2 oz turkey breast
½ cup crimini mushrooms, sliced

Dressing:
½ TBS extra virgin olive oil
½ TBS lemon juice
1 clove garlic, chopped (optional)
Salt and pepper to taste

Directions:

Combine all ingredients and toss with dressing ingredients. Dressing ingredients don't have to be combined separately before tossing.

Serves 1

Nutritional Profile							
Calories	409	Carbohydrates	28.40 g	Saturated Fat	3.65 g	Calcium	54.00 mg
Calories-Saturated Fat	33	Dietary Fiber	10.93 g	Fat - Total	24.10 g	Potassium	570.52 mg
Protein	26.29 g	Soluble Fiber	0.05 g	Cholesterol	47.06 mg	Sodium	400.85 mg

Mexican Cheese Salad

In this easy addition to your *Calorie-Lowering Plan*, enjoy the health-promoting anthocyanins found in black beans, which not only give them their beautiful dark coloration but provide you with protection against free radical activity.

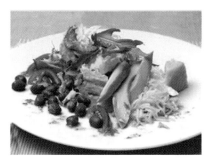

Ingredients:

4 cups romaine lettuce
1 cup cooked black or pinto beans (or half of 15-oz can, rinsed and drained)
¼ medium avocado, cubed
½ medium tomato, diced
1 oz-wt low-fat cheddar cheese, grated
2 TBS salsa
Juice from lime wedges, to taste
Salt and pepper to taste

Directions:

1.   Sprinkle beans, avocado, and tomato over greens.
2.   Top with cheddar cheese, your favorite salsa, and the juice of lime wedges.

Serves 1

Nutritional Profile							
Calories	392	Carbohydrates	55.67 g	Saturated Fat	2.19 g	Calcium	232.28 mg
Calories-Saturated Fat	20	Dietary Fiber	20.90 g	Fat - Total	9.23 g	Potassium	1469.43 mg
Protein	26.25 g	Soluble Fiber	4.13 g	Cholesterol	5.95 mg	Sodium	308.33 mg

Pineapple Chicken Salad

This unique combination of ingredients not only tastes great but the low-in-calorie pineapple provides you with an extra boost of vitamin C for added antioxidant protection and immune support.

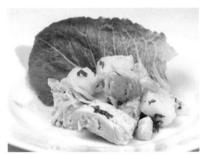

Photo shown with tumeric added

Ingredients:

1 cup diced pineapple
1 fennel bulb, sliced thin
¼ cup diced chicken breast
1 TBS extra virgin olive oil
½ TBS lemon juice
6 cups salad greens
Salt and pepper to taste

Directions:

Combine all ingredients except salad greens. Top salad greens with the Pineapple Chicken Salad mixture.

Serves 1

Nutritional Profile							
Calories	405	Carbohydrates	51.46 g	Sautrated Fat	2.37 g	Calcium	269.57 mg
Calories-Saturated Fat	21	Dietary Fiber	9.59 g	Fat - Total	17.26 g	Potassium	2789.90 mg
Protein	21.40 g	Soluble Fiber	0.01 g	Cholesterol	29.75 mg	Sodium	162.75 mg

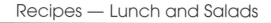

Romaine Salad with Goat Cheese and Mushrooms

Adding salmon or sardines to a *Calorie-Lowering Plan* is an easy way to help meet the recommended intake of those hard-to-find omega-3 fatty acids so important for optimal health.

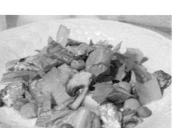

Photo shown without goat cheese and sunflower seeds

Ingredients:

1 oz-wt sardines or canned salmon
6 cups fresh romaine lettuce, chopped
½ cup sliced fresh crimini mushrooms
¼ cup frozen green peas, thawed
1 medium tomato, diced
1 ½ oz low fat soft goat cheese
1 TBS sunflower seeds

Dressing:
½ TBS extra virgin olive oil
1 clove garlic, chopped
1 tsp fresh lemon juice
Salt and pepper to taste

Directions:

Combine all ingredients and toss with dressing ingredients. Dressing ingredients don't have to be combined separately before tossing.

Serves 1

Nutritional Profile							
Calories	410	Carbohydrates	24.47 g	Saturated Fat	10.90 g	Calcium	321.87 mg
Calories-Saturated Fat	98	Dietary Fiber	9.95 g	Fat - Total	25.79 g	Potassium	1367.75 mg
Protein	24.70 g	Soluble Fiber	0.15 g	Cholesterol	47.07 mg	Sodium	388.67 mg

Tuna Salad Without Mayo

If you didn't think you could have
a tuna salad without mayo, try this
unique version that is low in calories
and still provides you with great taste.

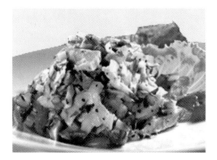

Ingredients:

3 oz light tuna packed in water, drained
1 clove garlic, chopped
½ TBS Dijon mustard
½ tsp honey
2 tsp fresh lemon juice
1 oz-wt soft silken tofu
¼ cup celery, chopped
4 olives, sliced
1 tsp sunflower seeds
½ medium avocado, diced
4 cups salad greens
Salt and pepper to taste

Directions:

1.   Chop garlic and let sit for 5 minutes to bring out its health-promoting
      properties.

2.   Combine all ingredients except avocado and salad greens.

3.   Place salad greens and avocado on a plate and top with the Tuna
      Without Mayo recipe.

Serves 1

Nutritional Profile							
Calories	354	Carbohydrates	25.14 g	Saturated Fat	2.06 g	Calcium	127.22 mg
Calories-Saturated Fat	19	Dietary Fiber	3.74 g	Fat - Total	16.42 g	Potassium	1722.86 mg
Protein	31.95 g	Soluble Fiber	0.02 g	Cholesterol	25.51 mg	Sodium	253.85 mg

Recipes
Dinner

Healthy Sautéed Scallops

Healthy Sauté your scallops and enjoy a great tasting dish without the use of heated oils that are not only unhealthy but add extra calories when trying to lose weight.

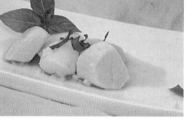

Ingredients:

3 oz-wt bay scallops or sea scallops
1 TBS low-sodium chicken or vegetable broth
1 medium clove garlic, chopped
½ tsp extra virgin olive oil
½ TBS fresh lemon juice
Salt and pepper to taste

Directions:

1. Chop garlic and let sit for 5 minutes to enhance its health-promoting benefits.
2. Heat 1 TBS broth over medium heat in a stainless steel skillet.
3. When broth begins to steam, add scallops and garlic and sauté for 2 minutes stirring frequently. After 2 minutes, turn scallops over and let cook on the other side for 1 minute. Scallops cook very quickly so watch your cooking time. Overcooked scallops become tough. (If you are using larger sea scallops, you'll need to cook for 1-2 minutes longer.)
4. Dress with extra virgin olive oil, lemon juice, garlic, salt and pepper.

Serves 1

Nutritional Profile							
Calories	94	Carbohydrates	3.52 g	Saturated Fat	0.41 g	Calcium	24.41 mg
Calories-Saturated Fat	4	Dietary Fiber	0.09 g	Fat - Total	2.97 g	Potassium	271.36 mg
Protein	13.06 g	Soluble Fiber	0.01 g	Cholesterol	24.95 mg	Sodium	124.55 mg

7-Minute Healthy Sautéed Chicken and Asparagus

Enjoy a rich source of protein and folate when you make this great-tasting chicken and asparagus *Calorie-Lowering* meal.

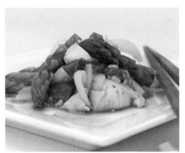

Photo shown with
onions and mustard added

Ingredients:

1 medium clove garlic, pressed
3 TBS chicken broth
6 oz-wt boneless, skinless chicken breast, cut into 1-inch pieces
3/4 lb asparagus, cut into 1-inch pieces (about 2 cups when cut)
1 tsp lemon juice
Pinch of red chili flakes
¼ TBS extra virgin olive oil
Salt and white pepper to taste

Directions:

1. Chop garlic and let sit for at least 5 minutes to bring out its hidden health benefits.
2. Heat 3 TBS broth in a stainless steel wok or 12-inch skillet. When broth begins to steam add chicken and cook for 3-4 minutes.
3. Add asparagus, lemon juice, and red chili flakes. Stir together and cover. Cook for another 2-3 minutes. This may have to cook for an extra couple minutes if the asparagus is thick. Toss with extra virgin olive oil. Season with salt and pepper to taste.

Serves 1

Nutritional Profile							
Calories	295	Carbohydrates	16.33 g	Saturated Fat	1.66 g	Calcium	96.43 mg
Calories-Saturated Fat	15	Dietary Fiber	7.40 g	Fat - Total	7.60 g	Potassium	1162.07 mg
Protein	42.27 g	Soluble Fiber	0.01 g	Cholesterol	93.98 mg	Sodium	89.13 mg

Black Bean Chili

A rich, hearty and flavorful vegetarian *Calorie-Lowering Plan* meal that is rich in nutrients and takes less than 30 minutes to prepare.

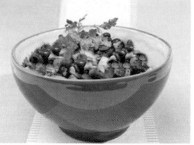

Ingredients:

½ medium onion, chopped
1 clove garlic, minced or pressed
1 cup cooked black beans (or half of 15 oz can black beans, rinsed)
½ - 15 oz can diced tomatoes
1 TBS chili powder
¼ cup cilantro

Directions:

1. Chop onions and mince or press garlic and let sit for at least 5 minutes to enhance their health-promoting properties.
2. Place all ingredients—except cilantro—in a pot, **cover**, and let simmer for about 20 minutes.
3. Top with cilantro and serve.

Serves 1

Nutritional Profile							
Calories	327	Carbohydrates	61.00 g	Saturated Fat	0.50 g	Calcium	119.18 mg
Calories-Saturated Fat	4	Dietary Fiber	20.28 g	Fat - Total	2.31 g	Potassium	854.46 mg
Protein	18.64 g	Soluble Fiber	4.13 g	Cholesterol	0 mg	Sodium	557.70 mg

Chicken Breast with Rosemary, Thyme and Sage

Herbs and spices are a great way to season almost any *Calorie-Lowering Plan* dish and only a few extra calories.

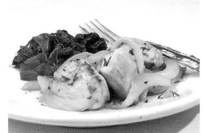

Photo shown with onions and mustard added

Ingredients:

1 clove garlic, chopped

1-½ oz-wt chicken breast, cut into cubes

½ TBS fresh lemon juice

2 cups organic low-fat chicken or vegetable broth

1 tsp fresh sage

1 tsp fresh thyme

1 tsp fresh rosemary

Salt and pepper to taste

Directions:

1. Chop garlic and let sit for 5 minutes to bring out its health-promoting properties.
2. Cut chicken and coat with lemon juice, salt, and pepper.
3. Heat broth and add chicken and herbs. Cook for 3-4 minutes until chicken is cooked through.

Serves 1

Nutritional Profile							
Calories	131	Carbohydrates	7.85 g	Saturated Fat	1.16 g	Calcium	38.77 mg
Calories-Saturated Fat	10	Dietary Fiber	0.30 g	Fat - Total	3.97 g	Potassium	517.19 mg
Protein	18.49 g	Soluble Fiber	0.01 g	Cholesterol	23.49 mg	Sodium	165.32 mg

Halibut with Ginger and Scallions

Add this delicious low-calorie Asian-flavored dish to your *Calorie-Lowering* menu. With plenty of protein and little fat, it's one of our favorites.

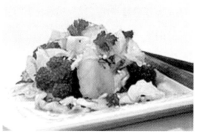

Photo shown with broccoli, cabbage and cilantro added

Ingredients:

2.5 oz-wt halibut

2 TBS low-sodium chicken or vegetable broth

½ TBS mirin rice wine*

1 medium clove garlic, chopped

¼ TBS tamari (soy sauce)

¼ TBS fresh lemon juice

¼ TBS minced fresh ginger

¼ cup coarsely chopped scallion

Salt and white pepper to taste

* Japanese rice cooking wine found in Asian section of market

Directions:

1. Chop garlic and let sit for 5 minutes to enhance its health-promoting properties

2. Bring the broth to a simmer on medium-high heat in a 10-inch skillet.

3. Add garlic, tamari, lemon juice, ginger, and scallions.

4. Place halibut on top, reduce heat to low and cover. Cook for about 5 minutes, depending on thickness. Season with salt and pepper. Remove steak and place on a plate. Spoon ginger and scallion mixture over fish and serve.

Serves 1

Nutritional Profile							
Calories	112	Carbohydrates	5.70 g	Saturated Fat	0.27 g	Calcium	56.63 mg
Calories-Saturated Fat	2	Dietary Fiber	0.76 g	Fat - Total	1.78 g	Potassium	427.34 mg
Protein	16.15 g	Soluble Fiber	0.21 g	Cholesterol	22.68 mg	Sodium	298.63 mg

Mediterranean Cod with Red Bell Peppers and Basil

Weight Loss Success is all about combining great taste with great nutrition and a minimal number of calories. This recipe is a winner on all three fronts.

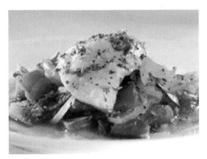

Ingredients:

½ medium onion, sliced thin
3 oz-wt cod fillets
2 TBS + ½ cup low-sodium chicken or vegetable broth
½ medium red bell pepper, diced
1 medium tomato, diced
½ TBS fresh basil, chopped
1 TBS fresh parsley, chopped
Salt and pepper to taste

Directions:

1. Slice onion and let sit for 5 minutes to bring out its health-promoting properties.
2. Heat 2 TBS broth in skillet. When broth begins to steam, add onions and bell pepper.
3. Add ½ cup broth, cod fillet, and tomato
4. Cover and cook over medium heat for 3-5 minutes or until fish is cooked.
5. Add chopped basil, parsley, and salt and pepper to taste.

Serves 1

Nutritional Profile							
Calories	138	Carbohydrates	14.72 g	Saturated Fat	0.31 g	Calcium	47.92 mg
Calories-Saturated Fat	3	Dietary Fiber	3.75 g	Fat - Total	1.47 g	Potassium	730.00 mg
Protein	17.33 g	Soluble Fiber	0 g	Cholesterol	32.28 mg	Sodium	81.18 mg

Miso Salmon

Among those fats that are important in the *Calorie-Lowering Plan* are the health-promoting omega-3 fatty acids, of which salmon is a great source. Enjoy this unique tasting salmon recipe that takes little time to prepare.

Photo shown served over shiitake mushrooms

Ingredients:

3 oz-wt salmon
½ TBS light miso
½ TBS Dijon mustard
1-½ tsp mirin rice wine*
½ tsp minced fresh ginger
½ tsp rice vinegar

* Japanese cooking rice wine found in Asian section of market

Directions:

1. Preheat broiler with rack in the middle of the oven. Place a stainless steel or cast iron skillet big enough to hold salmon under heat to get very hot (about 10 minutes).
2. Prepare glaze by mixing miso, Dijon mustard, mirin, ginger, and vinegar. Generously coat salmon with mixture.
3. Using a hot pad, pull pan away from heat and place salmon on hot pan, skin side down. Return to broiler. Keep in mind that it is cooking rapidly on both sides so it will be done very quickly, usually in 3–5 minutes depending on thickness. Test with a fork for doneness. It will flake easily when it is cooked. Salmon is best when it is still pink inside.

Serves 1

Nutritional Profile							
Calories	206	Carbohydrates	5.52 g	Saturated Fat	2.33 g	Calcium	21.00 mg
Calories-Saturated Fat	21	Dietary Fiber	0.21 g	Fat - Total	10.10 g	Potassium	369.22 mg
Protein	19.60 g	Soluble Fiber	0 g	Cholesterol	61.45 mg	Sodium	593.60 mg

Poached Halibut with Fennel and Cauliflower

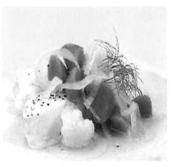

Calorie-Lowering Plan dishes taste so good you can share their great taste (and nutritional value) with your most finicky friends. This is among my favorites to serve to guests.

Ingredients:

¼ medium-sized onion, cut in half and sliced medium thick
2 oz-wt halibut, cut into small pieces
3/4 tsp fresh lemon juice
1 TBS + ½ cup chicken or vegetable broth
½ small carrot, sliced into ½-inch pieces
1/3 cup cauliflower florets, cut into quarters
¼ medium fennel bulb, sliced medium thick
1 medium clove garlic, pressed
Salt and pepper to taste
Chopped fennel green tops for garnish

Directions:

1. Slice onion and chop garlic and let sit for at least 5 minutes to bring out their hidden health-promoting properties.
2. Rub halibut with lemon juice and season with a little salt and pepper. Set aside.
3. Heat 1 TBS broth in a 12-inch stainless steel skillet Healthy Sauté onion in broth over medium heat for 5 minutes stirring frequently.
4. Add rest of broth and carrots. Simmer on medium heat for about 10 minutes covered.
5. Add cauliflower, fennel, and garlic. Place halibut on top and continue to cook covered for about 6 more minutes. Season with salt and pepper.
6. Serve halibut with vegetables and broth. Sprinkle with chopped fennel greens.

Serves 1

Nutritional Profile							
Calories	126	Carbohydrates	12,.85 g	Saturated Fat	0.35 g	Calcium	84.11 mg
Calories-Saturated Fat	3	Dietary Fiber	3.84 g	Fat - Total	2.09 g	Potassium	743.95 mg
Protein	15.28 g	Soluble Fiber	0.55 g	Cholesterol	18.14 mg	Sodium	105.64 mg

Quick Broiled Salmon with Ginger Mint Salsa

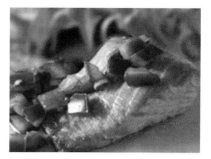

Variety is an important part of *Weight Loss Success.* This great-tasting salsa is especially good served on salmon.

Ingredients:

2-½ oz-wt salmon fillet
1 tsp lemon juice
Salt and pepper to taste
Extra virgin olive oil, to taste

Salsa
½ ripe tomato, diced
¼ cup green onions, minced
½ tsp ginger, minced

1 tsp fresh mint, minced
½ tsp lime juice
Salt and pepper to taste

Directions:

1. Preheat broiler and place an all stainless steel skillet (be sure the handle is also stainless steel) or cast iron pan under the heat for about 10 minutes to get it very hot. The pan should be 5 to 7 inches from the heat source.
2. Rub salmon with 1 tsp fresh lemon juice, salt and pepper. (You can Quick Broil with the skin on; it just takes a minute or two longer. The skin will peel right off after cooking.)
3. Using a hot pad, pull pan away from heat and place salmon on hot pan, skin side down. Return to broiler. Keep in mind that it is cooking rapidly on both sides so it will be done very quickly, usually in 3–5 minutes depending on thickness. Test with a fork for doneness. It will flake easily when it is cooked. Salmon is best when it is still pink inside.
4. While the salmon is cooking, combine all salsa ingredients.
5. When salmon is ready, spoon salsa over salmon.
6. Garnish with mint and a sprinkle of extra virgin olive oil

Serves 1

Nutritional Profile							
Calories	161	Carbohydrates	5.21 g	Saturated Fat	1.96 g	Calcium	43.80 mg
Calories-Saturated Fat	18	Dietary Fiber	1.17 g	Fat - Total	8.19 g	Potassium	523.73 mg
Protein	16.60 g	Soluble Fiber	0.27 g	Cholesterol	51.21 mg	Sodium	47.31 mg

Salmon with Dill Sauce

A classic dish that offers great taste and nutrition to your *Calorie-Lowering Plan*. Salmon is one of the best sources of those hard-to-come-by omega-3 fatty acids. Enjoy!

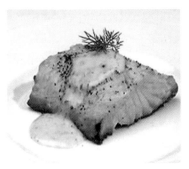

Ingredients:

3 oz-wt salmon fillet, cut in half
1 + ½ tsp lemon juice
Salt and pepper to taste

Dill Sauce
2 oz low-fat plain yogurt
½ medium cucumber, seeded and diced
½ TBS fresh dill weed, chopped
Salt and pepper to taste

Directions:

1. Preheat broiler on high and place an all stainless steel skillet (be sure the handle is also stainless steel) or cast iron pan under the heat for about 10 minutes to get it very hot. The pan should be 5 to 7 inches from the heat source.
2. Rub salmon with 1 tsp lemon juice, salt and pepper. (You can Quick Broil with the skin on; it just takes a minute or two longer. The skin will peel right off after cooking.)
3. Using a hot pad, pull pan away from heat and place salmon on hot pan, skin side down. Return to broiler. Keep in mind that it is cooking rapidly on both sides so it will be done very quickly, usually in 3–5 minutes depending on thickness. Test with a fork for doneness. It will flake easily when it is cooked. Salmon is best when it is still pink inside. After salmon is cooked, sprinkle it with remaining 1 tsp lemon juice.
4. Top salmon with dill sauce.

Serves 1

5 Nutritional Profile							
Calories	258	Carbohydrates	15.63 g	Saturated Fat	2.97 g	Calcium	393.03 mg
Calories-Saturated Fat	27	Dietary Fiber	5.73 g	Fat - Total	11.01 g	Potassium	1527.23 mg
Protein	28.29 g	Soluble Fiber	1.26 g	Cholesterol	64.85 mg	Sodium	205.56 mg

Salmon with Mustard

Mustard adds a tangy flavor to omega-3 rich salmon—a great combination to add to your *Calorie-Lowering Plan* menu.

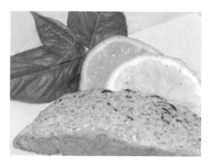

Ingredients:

5 oz-wt salmon fillet, cut in half
1 tsp lemon juice
Salt and pepper to taste
½ TBS Dijon mustard

Directions:

1. Preheat broiler and place an all stainless steel skillet (be sure the handle is also stainless steel) or cast iron pan under the heat for about 10 minutes to get it very hot. The pan should be 5 to 7 inches from the heat source.

2. Rub salmon with fresh lemon juice, salt and pepper and spread Dijon mustard on fillets before broiling. (You can Quick Broil with the skin on; it just takes a minute or two longer. The skin will peel right off after cooking.)

3. Using a hot pad, pull pan away from heat and place salmon on hot pan, skin side down. Return to broiler. Keep in mind that it is cooking rapidly on both sides so it will be done very quickly, in about 5 minutes. Test with a fork for doneness. It will flake easily when it is cooked. Salmon is best when it is still pink inside. Cooking time is based on 10 minutes for every inch of thickness.

Serves 1

Nutritional Profile							
Calories	169	Carbohydrates	2.38 g	Saturated Fat	2.27 g	Calcium	17.58 mg
Calories-Saturated Fat	20	Dietary Fiber	0.04 g	Fat - Total	10.39 g	Potassium	316.83 mg
Protein	15.53 g	Soluble Fiber	0.02 g	Cholesterol	51.21 mg	Sodium	216.25 mg

Seared Asian Tuna

Rich in B-vitamins, selenium, and protein, this nutrient-rich and flavorful Asian-inspired dish can be prepared in a matter of minutes.

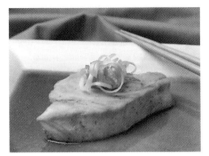

Ingredients:

2.5 oz-wt tuna
1 TBS mirin rice wine*
½ + ½ TBS fresh squeezed lemon juice
1 TBS tamari (soy sauce)
½ TBS minced fresh ginger
3 TBS minced scallion
Salt and white pepper to taste

* Japanese cooking rice wine found in Asian section of market

Directions:

1.   Preheat 10-12 inch stainless steel skillet over medium-high heat for 2 minutes.
2.   While pan is preheating, rub tuna with ½ TBS lemon juice, season with a little salt and white pepper, and prepare ginger and scallion.
3.   Place tuna on preheated skillet and cook for 1-2 minutes on each side, depending on thickness, and then remove from skillet. Seared tuna is best when medium rare.
4.   Turn heat down to medium and add rest of ingredients to pan in order given, and cook for 1 minute. Season with salt and pepper. Pour over tuna and serve.

Serves 1

Nutritional Profile							
Calories	98	Carbohydrates	3.57 g	Saturated Fat	0.18 g	Calcium	29.45 mg
Calories-Saturated Fat	2	Dietary Fiber	0.72 g	Fat - Total	0.75 g	Potassium	426.49 mg
Protein	18.89 g	Soluble Fiber	0.16 g	Cholesterol	31.89 mg	Sodium	1035.17 mg

Spicy Asian Shrimp

Shrimp is a rich source of vitamin D —a vitamin which has been receiving increasing notoriety of late, especially for its importance in bone health. This recipe is not only low in calories, but will get you a long way to meet the daily requirements for vitamin D.

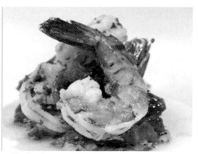

Photo shown served on bed of tomatoes

Ingredients:

1 medium garlic clove, chopped
3 oz-wt medium-sized shrimp, peeled and deveined
1 TBS + ½ TBS fresh lemon juice
Salt and pepper to taste
3 TBS low-sodium chicken or vegetable broth
pinch of red pepper flakes
2 TBS orange juice
½ TBS minced fresh ginger
¼ TBS extra virgin olive oil

Directions:

1. Chop garlic and let sit for 5 minutes to enhance its health-promoting properties.
2. Peel and devein shrimp.
3. Rub shrimp with 1 TBS lemon juice, salt and pepper.
4. Heat 3 TBS broth over medium-low heat in a stainless steel skillet.
5. When broth begins to steam, add shrimp, red pepper flakes, orange juice, and ginger and sauté. Stir frequently. After 2 minutes, turn the shrimp over and add garlic. Sauté until shrimp are pink and opaque throughout (approximately 3 minutes). Shrimp cook quickly, so watch your cooking time. They become tough if overcooked.
6. Dress with the extra virgin olive oil and the remaining 1 TBS lemon juice.

Serves 1

Nutritional Profile							
Calories	148	Carbohydrates	7.17 g	Saturated Fat	0.84 g	Calcium	55.68 mg
Calories-Saturated Fat	8	Dietary Fiber	0.28 g	Fat - Total	5.23 g	Potassium	284.35 mg
Protein	18.26 g	Soluble Fiber	0.05 g	Cholesterol	129.27 mg	Sodium	134.02 mg

Thai Scallops (or Shrimp) with Basil

Rich in nutrients and flavor, this Thai inspired *Weight Loss Success* dish is hard to beat.

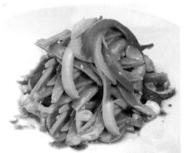

Photo shown with
carrots and without shellfish

Ingredients:

3/4 cup low-sodium chicken or vegetable broth

1 cup green beans, cut into1-inch lengths

½ cup fresh sliced red bell peppers, sliced

½ tsp grated ginger

1 clove garlic

2 TBS coconut milk

½ tsp Thai curry paste

2 oz-wt medium raw shrimp or scallops

2 TBS fresh basil, chopped

¼ cup sunflower seeds

Directions:

1. Healthy sauté green beans in 3 TBS broth for 3 minutes covered.
2. Add bell peppers and sauté for an additional 3 minutes covered.
3. Add 1 tsp Thai curry paste, garlic, ginger and coconut milk. Simmer for 3-5 minutes.
4. Add shrimp, basil, and sunflower seeds and cook for another 3 minutes uncovered.

Serves 1

Nutritional Profile							
Calories	411	Carbohydrates	32.75 g	Saturated Fat	7.84 g	Calcium	503.95 mg
Calories-Saturated Fat	71	Dietary Fiber	16.23 g	Fat - Total	19.86 g	Potassium	1233.85 mg
Protein	30.35 g	Soluble Fiber	3.27 g	Cholesterol	30.05 mg	Sodium	246.72 mg

Recipes
Side Vegetables and Dips

1-Minute Spinach 1

Enjoy this quick and easy addition to your *Calorie-Lowering Plan* that provides you with a rich source of health-promoting nutrients such as vitamin A,K, C, as well as manganese and folate.

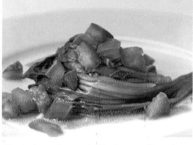

Photo shown topped with chopped tomatoes

Ingredients:

1 medium fresh garlic, pressed
     or chopped
½ lb fresh spinach
½ tsp lemon juice
½ tsp extra virgin olive oil
Salt and cracked black pepper to taste
Optional: chopped tomato
½ tsp tamari
1 TBS goat cheese
1 TBS sesame seeds

Directions:

1.   Chop or press garlic and let it sit for 5 minutes to bring out its health promoting benefits.
2.   Bring lightly salted water to a rapid boil in a large pot.
3.   Cut stems off spinach leaves and clean well. This can be done easily by leaving spinach bundled and cutting off stems all at once. **Rinse spinach leaves very well as they often contain a lot of soil.**
4.   Cook spinach for 1 minute after water returns to a boil.
5.   Drain and press out excess water. Toss in rest of ingredients while spinach is still hot. For best taste cut into small pieces before serving.

Serves 1

Nutritional Profile							
Calories	76	Carbohydrates	9.17 g	Saturated Fat	0.48 g	Calcium	227.6 mg
Calories-Saturated Fat	4	Dietary Fiber	5.04 g	Fat - Total	3.23 g	Potassium	1277.86 mg
Protein	6.6 g	Soluble Fiber	0.01 g	Cholesterol	0 mg	Sodium	179.48 mg

1-Minute Spinach 2

Enjoy this quick and easy addition to your *Calorie-Lowering Plan* that provides you with a rich source of healthy promoting nutrients such as vitamin A,K, C, as well as manganese and folate.

Photo shown topped with chopped tomatoes

Ingredients:

1 medium fresh garlic, pressed
or chopped
1 lbs fresh spinach
½ tsp lemon juice

Salt and cracked black pepper to taste
Optional: chopped tomato

Directions:

1.   Chop or press garlic and let it sit for 5 minutes to bring out its health-promoting benefits.
2.   Bring lightly salted water to a rapid boil in a large pot.
3.   Cut stems off spinach leaves and clean well. This can be done easily by leaving spinach bundled and cutting off stems all at once. **Rinse spinach leaves very well as they often contain a lot of soil.**
4.   Cook spinach for 1 minute after water returns to a boil.
5.   Drain and press out excess water. For best taste cut into small pieces before serving.

Serves 1

Nutritional Profile							
Calories	107	Carbohydrates	17.18 g	Saturated Fat	0.29 g	Calcium	451,95 mg
Calories-Saturated Fat	3	Dietary Fiber	10.02 g	Fat - Total	1.78 g	Potassium	2540.21 mg
Protein	13.08 g	Soluble Fiber	0 g	Cholesterol	0 mg	Sodium	358.62 mg

1-Minute Spinach 3

Enjoy this quick and easy addition to your *Calorie-Lowering Plan* that provides you with a rich source of healthy promoting nutrients such as vitamin A,K, C, as well as manganese and folate.

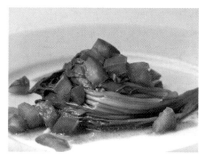

Photo shown topped with chopped tomatoes

Ingredients:

1 medium fresh garlic, pressed or- chopped
½ lb fresh spinach
½ tsp lemon juice
Salt and cracked black pepper to taste
Optional: chopped tomato

Directions:

1. Chop or press garlic and let it sit for 5 minutes to bring out its health-promoting benefits.
2. Bring lightly salted water to a rapid boil in a large pot.
3. Cut stems off spinach leaves and clean well. This can be done easily by leaving spinach bundled and cutting off stems all at once. Rinse spinach leaves very well as they often contain a lot of soil.
4. Cook spinach for 1 minute after water returns to boil.
5. Drain and press out excess water. Toss in rest of ingredients while spinach is still hot. For best taste cut into small pieces before serving.

Serves 1

Nutritional Profile							
Calories	55	Carbohydrates	8.95 g	Saturated Fat	0.14 g	Calcium	227.42 mg
Calories-Saturated Fat	1	Dietary Fiber	5.03 g	Fat - Total	0.89 g	Potassium	1274.71 mg
Protein	6.59 g	Soluble Fiber	0 g	Cholesterol	0 mg	Sodium	179.45 mg

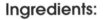

3-Minute Guacamole

Guacamole is very popular in Mexico and Southwestern cuisines. It only takes 3 minutes to add this easy version to your *Calorie-Lowering Plan* and get an extra boost of vitamins A, C, and K.

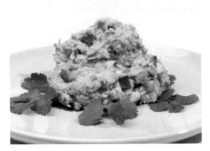

Photo shown with tomatoes added

Ingredients:

¼ medium avocado
½ TBS lemon juice
¼ cup fresh cilantro leaves
Salt and pepper to taste

Directions:

Mash avocado with a fork and combine with remaining ingredients.

Serves 1

Nutritional Profile							
Calories	83	Carbohydrates	4.96 g	Saturated Fat	1.07 g	Calcium	6.83 mg
Calories-Saturated Fat	10	Dietary Fiber	3.41 g	Fat - Total	7.37 g	Potassium	255.25 mg
Protein	1.04 g	Soluble Fiber	0.01 g	Cholesterol	0 mg	Sodium	3.78 mg

3-Minute Swiss Chard 1

Swiss chard is one of the most nutrient-rich foods to add to your *Calorie-Lowering Plan*. It's a great source of vitamins A, C, K, magnesium, and manganese, and a complement to almost any of your favorite meals.

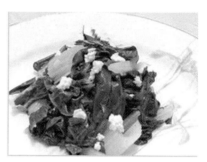

Photo shown served with goat cheese

Ingredients:

1 medium clove garlic, chopped or pressed
½ lb Swiss chard, chopped
1 medium clove garlic, chopped or pressed
½ tsp extra virgin olive oil
½ tsp lemon juice
Optional: ½ tsp tamari, 1 TBS feta cheese
Salt and black pepper to taste

Directions:

1.   Chop or press garlic and let sit for 5 minutes to bring out its health-promoting properties.
2.   Fill a large pot (3 quart) with lots of water. Make sure water is at a rapid boil before adding Swiss chard.
3.   Cut off tough bottom part of Swiss chard stems.
4.   Chop leaves and then add them to the boiling water. Do not cover. Cook for 3 minutes after water returns to boil.
5.   Carefully remove chard from water, place in colander and press out excess water.
6.   Transfer to serving dish and toss with lemon juice, olive oil, salt and pepper. For best taste cut into small pieces before serving.

Serves 1

Nutritional Profile							
Calories	66	Carbohydrates	9.20 g	Saturated Fat	0.40 g	Calcium	118.56 mg
Calories-Saturated Fat	4	Dietary Fiber	3.67 g	Fat - Total	2.79 g	Potassium	868.72 mg
Protein	4.19 g	Soluble Fiber	0 g	Cholesterol	0 mg	Sodium	483.36 mg

3-Minute Swiss Chard 2

Swiss chard is one of the most nutrient-rich foods to add to your *Calorie-Lowering Plan*. It's a great source of vitamins A, C, K, magnesium, and manganese, and a complement to almost any of your favorite meals.

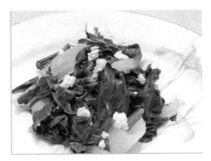

Photo shown served with goat cheese

Ingredients:

½ lb Swiss chard, chopped
1 medium clove garlic, chopped or pressed
½ tsp lemon juice
Salt and black pepper to taste

Directions:

1.   Chop or press garlic and let sit for 5 minutes to bring out its health-promoting properties.
2.   Fill a large pot (3 quart) with lots of water. Make sure water is at a rapid boil before adding Swiss chard.
3.   Cut off tough bottom part of Swiss chard stems.
4.   Chop leaves and then add them to the boiling water. Do not cover. Cook for 3 minutes after water returns to a boil.
5.   Carefully remove chard from water, place in colander and press out excess water.
6.   Transfer to serving dish and toss with lemon juice, salt and pepper. For best taste cut into small pieces before serving.

Serves 1

Nutritional Profile							
Calories	46	Carbohydrates	9.2 g	Saturated Fat	0.07 g	Calcium	118.56 mg
Calories-Saturated Fat	1	Dietary Fiber	3.67 g	Fat - Total	0.46 g	Potassium	868.74 mg
Protein	4.19 g	Soluble Fiber	0 g	Cholesterol	0 mg	Sodium	483.36 mg

5-Minute Broccoli 1

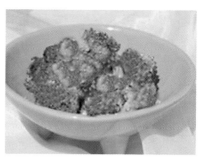

Broccoli, like other cruciferous vegetables, adds not only a rich source of vitamins A, C, K, and folate to your *Calorie-Lowering Plan*, but health-promoting sulfur compounds that help your liver detoxify potentially toxic substances.

Ingredients:

½ lb broccoli
1 clove garlic, chopped or pressed
¼ TBS extra virgin olive oil
1 tsp lemon juice
Salt and pepper to taste
Optional ingredients: ½ TBS feta cheese or sliced kalamata olives

Directions:

1. Fill the bottom of the steamer with 2 inches of water.
2. While steam is building up in steamer, cut broccoli florets into quarters. Peel stems and cut into ¼-inch pieces. Let florets and stems sit for 5 minutes to bring out their hidden health benefits.
3. Chop or press garlic and let sit for at least 5 minutes.
4. If you are cooking stems, steam for 2 minutes before adding the florets. Steam florets for 5 minutes
5. Transfer to a bowl. Toss broccoli with the remaining ingredients while it is still hot.

Serves 1

Nutritional Profile							
Calories	113	Carbohydrates	16.49 g	Saturated Fat	0.59 g	Calcium	112.38 mg
Calories-Saturated Fat	5	Dietary Fiber	5.98 g	Fat - Total	4.35 g	Potassium	735.01 mg
Protein	6.61 g	Soluble Fiber	0.55 g	Cholesterol	0 mg	Sodium	75.40 mg

5-Minute Broccoli 2

Broccoli, like other cruciferous vegetables, adds not only a rich source of vitamins A, C, K, and folate to your *Calorie-Lowering Plan*, but health-promoting sulfur compounds that help your liver detoxify potentially toxic substances.

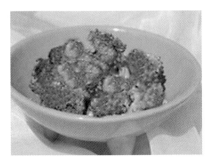

Ingredients:

1 lbs broccoli
1 medium clove garlic, chopped or pressed
¼ TBS extra virgin olive oil
1 tsp lemon juice
Salt and pepper to taste
Optional ingredients: ½ TBS feta cheese or sliced kalamata olives

Directions:

1. Fill the bottom of the steamer with 2 inches of water.
2. While steam is building up in steamer, cut broccoli florets into quarters. Peel stems and cut into ¼-inch pieces. Let florets and stems sit for 5 minutes to bring out their hidden health benefits.
3. Chop or press garlic and let sit for at least 5 minutes.
4. If you are cooking stems, steam for 2 minutes before adding the florets. Steam florets for 5 minutes.
5. Transfer to a bowl. For more flavor, toss broccoli with the remaining ingredients while it is still hot.

Serves 1

Nutritional Profile							
Calories	190	Carbohydrates	31.55 g	Saturated Fat	0.68 g	Calcium	218.97 mg
Calories-Saturated Fat	6	Dietary Fiber	11.88 g	Fat - Total	5.19 g	Potassium	1451.69 mg
Protein	13.00 g	Soluble Fiber	1.10 g	Cholesterol	0 mg	Sodium	150.25 mg

5-Minute Brussels Sprouts with Mustard

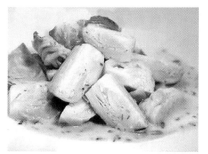

Even if you have not been a fan of Brussels sprouts, I think you will love adding this recipe to your *Weight Loss Success* menu. Like their cousins broccoli and kale, they are rich in health-promoting sulfur compounds, which help cenhance liver. And they only take minutes to prepare. Enjoy!

Ingredients:
½ lb Brussels sprouts
1 medium clove garlic, chopped or pressed
¼ TBS extra virgin olive oil
½ tsp lemon juice
½ TBS Dijon mustard
½ tsp honey
Salt and black pepper to taste

Directions:
1. Fill the bottom of the steamer with 2 inches of water.
2. While steam is building up in steamer, cut Brussels sprouts into quarters and let sit for at least 5 minutes to bring out their hidden health benefits.
3. Chop or press garlic and let sit for at least 5 minutes to bring out their health-promoting properties.
4. Steam Brussels sprouts for 5 minutes.
5. While sprouts are cooking combine the rest of the ingredients in a small bowl and mix well.
6. Transfer Brussels sprouts to the big bowl and toss with mustard mixture.

Serves 2

Nutritional Profile							
Calories	151	Carbohydrates	25.89 g	Saturated Fat	0.64 g	Calcium	101.07 mg
Calories-Saturated Fat	6	Dietary Fiber	8.70 g	Fat - Total	4.20 g	Potassium	899.24 mg
Protein	7.88 g	Soluble Fiber	4.55 g	Cholesterol	0 mg	Sodium	237.37 mg

5-Minute Cauliflower with Turmeric

The turmeric in this recipe not only adds great flavor but added anti-inflammatory protection to your *Calorie-Lowering Plan.*

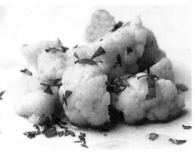

Ingredients:

½ lb cauliflower
1 medium clove garlic, pressed or chopped
5 TBS low-sodium chicken or vegetable broth
½ tsp turmeric
¼ TBS extra virgin olive oil
1 tsp lemon juice
Salt and pepper to taste

Directions:

1. Cut cauliflower florets into quarters and let sit for 5 minutes to bring out their hidden health benefits.
2. Press or chop garlic and let sit for 5 minutes.
3. Heat 2-½ TBS broth in a stainless steel skillet on medium heat.
4. When broth begins to steam, add cauliflower. Sprinkle turmeric on top of cauliflower and cover. Cook for no more than 5 minutes.
5. Transfer to a bowl. For more flavor, toss cauliflower with the remaining ingredients while it is still hot.

Serves 1

Nutritional Profile							
Calories	102	Carbohydrates	13.87 g	Saturated Fat	0.75 g	Calcium	59.19 mg
Calories-Saturated Fat	6	Dietary Fiber	4.85 g	Fat - Total	4.48 g	Potassium	756.48 mg
Protein	5.40 g	Soluble Fiber	1.64 g	Cholesterol	0 mg	Sodium	80.27 mg

5-Minute Collard Greens 1

Collard greens are one of the best plant-based sources of calcium — almost as much as a cup of milk with half the calories and almost no fat! It's no wonder they are a great addition to your *Calorie-Lowering Plan.*

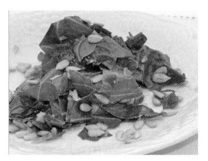

Photo shown served with sunflower seeds

Ingredients:

½ lbs collard greens cut into 1/8" slices
1 medium clove garlic, chopped or pressed
½ TBS extra virgin olive oil
½ tsp lemon juice
1 clove garlic, chopped
Salt and pepper to taste

Directions:

1.   Fill the bottom of the steamer with 2 inches of water.
2.   While steam is building up in steamer, chop collard greens and let sit for 5 minutes to bring out their hidden health benefits.
3.   Chop or press garlic and let sit for at least 5 minutes.
4.   Steam greens for 5 minutes.
5.   Transfer to a bowl. For more flavor, cut greens into small pieces and toss with the remaining ingredients while they are still hot.

Serves 1

Nutritional Profile							
Calories	130	Carbohydrates	13.62 g	Saturated Fat	1.13 g	Calcium	331.75 mg
Calories-Saturated Fat	10	Dietary Fiber	8.21 g	Fat - Total	7.96 g	Potassium	392.45 mg
Protein	5.66 g	Soluble Fiber	3.27 g	Cholesterol	0 mg	Sodium	45.64 mg

5-Minute Collard Greens 2

Collard greens are one of the best plant-based sources of calcium — almost as much as a cup of milk with half the calories and almost no fat! It's no wonder they are a great addition to your *Calorie-Lowering Plan.*

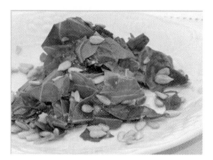

Photo shown served with sunflower seeds

Ingredients:

½ lbs collard greens cut into 1/8" slices
1 medium clove garlic, chopped or pressed
½ TBS extra virgin olive oil
½ tsp lemon juice
1 clove garlic, chopped
Salt and pepper to taste

Directions:

1. Fill the bottom of the steamer with 2 inches of water.
2. While steam is building up in steamer, chop collard greens and let sit for 5 minutes to bring out their hidden health benefits.
3. Chop or press garlic and let sit for at least 5 minutes.
4. Steam greens for 5 minutes.
5. Transfer to a bowl. For more flavor, cut greens into small pieces and toss with the remaining ingredients while they are still hot.

Serves 1

Nutritional Profile							
Calories	71	Carbohydrates	13.62 g	Saturated Fat	0.13 g	Calcium	331.75 mg
Calories-Saturated Fat	1	Dietary Fiber	8.21 g	Fat - Total	0.96 g	Potassium	392.45 mg
Protein	5.66 g	Soluble Fiber	3.27 g	Cholesterol	0 mg	Sodium	45.64 mg

5-Minute Italian Kale

With this delicious, easy-to-prepare recipe you can include kale as part of your *Calorie-Lowering Plan* in a matter of minutes. Kale is one of the healthiest vegetables around with one serving providing you with an excellent source of health-promoting vitamins A and E. Enjoy!

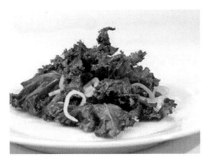

Photo shown with onions

Ingredients:

½ pound Italian (Lacinato) kale (or any variety) sliced 1/8" thick
1 medium clove garlic, pressed or chopped
1 tsp lemon juice
¼ TBS extra virgin olive oil
Salt and black pepper to taste
Optional: 1 medium onion

Directions:

1. Chop garlic and let sit for 5 minutes to enhance its health-promoting properties.
2. Fill bottom of steamer with 2 inches of water and bring to boil.
3. While water is coming to a boil, slice kale leaves into 1/8" inch slices. Let kale sit for at least 5 minutes to bring out it health-promoting properties.
4. When water comes to a boil, add kale to the steamer basket and cover. Steam for 5 minutes.
5. Transfer to a bowl For more flavor cut greens into small pieces and toss withthe remaining ingredients while it is still hot.

Serves 1

Nutritional Profile							
Calories	147	Carbohydrates	23.64 g	Saturated Fat	0.71 g	Calcium	309.25 mg
Calories-Saturated Fat	6	Dietary Fiber	4.59 g	Fat - Total	5.10 g	Potassium	1026.10 mg
Protein	7.60 g	Soluble Fiber	1.82 g	Cholesterol	0 mg	Sodium	97.83 mg

5-Minute Mediterranean Medley

This is a perfect way to prepare a variety of vegetables and add more nutrition to your *Calorie-Lowering Plan* in the same amount of time it takes to cook just one. Use this technique to cook an array of your favorite vegetables.

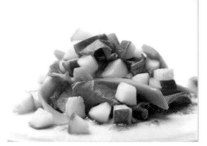

Photo shown with zucchini in place of broccoli

Ingredients:

1-½ cups broccoli florets, cut into quarters
1-½ cups kale, chopped
½ medium carrot, sliced
1 clove garlic, chopped or pressed
½ TBS extra virgin olive oil
1 tsp lemon juice
Salt and pepper to taste

Directions:

1. Fill the bottom of the steamer with 2 inches of water.
2. While steam is building up in steamer, cut broccoli, and chop kale and let sit for at least 5 minutes to bring out its hidden health benefits.
3. Slice carrots ¼ inch thick.
4. Chop or press garlic and let sit for at least 5 minutes to bring out its health-promoting properties.
5. Steam broccoli, kale, and carrots for 5 minutes.
6. Transfer to a bowl. Toss vegetables, while they are still hot, with garlic and the rest of the ingredients.

Serves 1

Nutritional Profile							
Calories	158	Carbohydrates	19.99 g	Saturated Fat	1.16 g	Calcium	202.65 mg
Calories-Saturated Fat	10	Dietary Fiber	6.14 g	Fat - Total	8.16 g	Potassium	911.29 mg
Protein	6.98 g	Soluble Fiber	1.52 g	Cholesterol	0 mg	Sodium	93.58 mg

Garlic Dip

This recipe makes a great appetizer before dinner or a snack any time of the day, Garlic not only has wonderful flavor but adds extra antibacterial and antioxidant protection to your *Calorie-Lowering* menu.

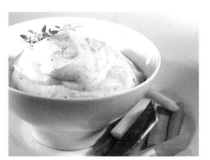

Ingredients:

2 cups cooked or 1-15-oz can (no-BPA) garbanzo beans
1 TBS lemon juice
3 medium cloves garlic, chopped
¼ cup chicken or vegetable broth
2 TBS extra virgin olive oil
Salt and pepper to taste

Directions:

Combine all ingredients in a blender and blend until smooth. Serve with your favorite crudités.

Serves 8

Nutritional Profile							
Calories	101	Carbohydrates	11.87 g	Saturated Fat	0.62 g	Calcium	22.56 mg
Calories-Saturated Fat	6	Dietary Fiber	3.15 g	Fat - Total	4.61 g	Potassium	132.63 mg
Protein	3.86 g	Soluble Fiber	0.97 g	Cholesterol	0 mg	Sodium	5.33 mg

Healthy Mashed Sweet Potatoes

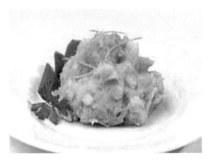

This full-flavored sweet potato dish is quick and easy to prepare and makes a healthy and unique addition to your *Calorie-Lowering Plan*. In fact, one serving of this recipe contains only 85 calories but provides over 200% of your daily value (DV) for vitamin A. Enjoy!

Ingredients:

½ medium-sized sweet potato or yam, peeled and sliced thin for quick cooking
½ TBS fresh orange juice
¼ TBS extra virgin olive oil
Salt and white pepper to taste

Directions:

1. Bring lightly salted water to a boil in a steamer with a tight fitting lid.
2. Steam peeled and sliced sweet potatoes in steamer basket, covered, for about 10 minutes, or until tender.
3. Mash with potato masher, adding rest of ingredients.

Serves 1

Nutritional Profile							
Calories	85	Carbohydrates	12.61 g	Saturated Fat	0.52 g	Calcium	22.51 mg
Calories-Saturated Fat	5	Dietary Fiber	1.90 g	Fat - Total	3.60 g	Potassium	286.25 mg
Protein	1.20 g	Soluble Fiber	0 g	Cholesterol	0 mg	Sodium	20.6 mg

Healthy Sautéed Crimini Mushrooms 1

Enjoy this easy-to-prepare recipe that complements many of your favorite dishes and is a great addition to your *Calorie-Lowering Plan*. You will also be enjoying a rich source of health-promoting selenium, vitamin B12, and copper along with the great flavor of crimini mushrooms.

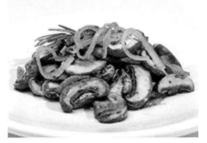

Photo shown with onions

Ingredients:

3 TBS low-sodium chicken or vegetable broth
½ lb crimini mushrooms, sliced
½ TBS extra virgin olive oil
Salt and pepper to taste

Directions:

1.   Heat 3 TBS broth over medium heat in a stainless steel skillet.
2.   When broth begins to steam, add the sliced mushrooms, cover, and sauté for 3 minutes. They will release liquid as they cook. Uncover and stir constantly for the last 4 minutes as crimini mushrooms are not as watery as other button mushrooms. The liquid will evaporate, and the mushrooms will become golden brown but not burned.
3.   For best flavor toss with olive oil, salt, and pepper while still hot.

Serves 1

Nutritional Profile							
Calories	114	Carbohydrates	10.02 g	Saturated Fat	1.07 g	Calcium	41.72 mg
Calories-Saturated Fat	10	Dietary Fiber	1.36 g	Fat - Total	7.36 g	Potassium	1036.40 mg
Protein	6.12 g	Soluble Fiber	0 g	Cholesterol	0 mg	Sodium	20.36 mg

Healthy Sautéed Crimini Mushrooms 2

Enjoy this easy-to-prepare recipe that complements many of your favorite dishes and is a great addition to your *Calorie-Lowering Plan*. You will also be enjoying a rich source of health-promoting selenium, vitamin B12, and copper along with the great flavor of crimini mushrooms.

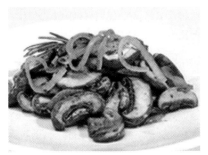

Photo shown with onions

Ingredients:

¼ lb crimini mushrooms, sliced
3 TBS low-sodium chicken or vegetable broth
Salt and pepper to taste

Directions:

1. Heat 3 TBS broth over medium heat in a stainless steel skillet.
2. When broth begins to steam, add the sliced mushrooms, cover, and sauté for 3 minutes. They will release liquid as they cook. Uncover and stire constantly for the last 4 minutes as crimini mushrooms are not as watery as other button mushrooms. The liquid will evaporate, and the mushrooms will become golden brown but not burned.
3. Add salt and pepper to taste.

Serves 1

Nutritional Profile							
Calories	29	Carbohydrates	5.15 g	Saturated Fat	0.06 g	Calcium	21.31 mg
Calories-Saturated Fat	1	Dietary Fiber	0.68 g	Fat - Total	0.25 g	Potassium	527.37 mg
Protein	3.28 g	Soluble Fiber	0 g	Cholesterol	0 mg	Sodium	13.55 mg

Healthy Sautéed Shiitake Mushrooms

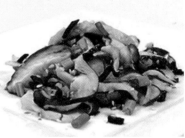

Long enjoyed in Asia for their health-promoting benefits, we now know that they are a good source or iron and protein as well s special health-promoting compounds that have cholesterol-lowering and immune stimulating properties. Enjoy them as part of your *Calorie-Lowering Plan* as a complement to both fish and poultry dishes.

Ingredients:

1 medium clove garlic, chopped or pressed
½ lb fresh sliced shiitake mushrooms
3 TBS low-sodium chicken or vegetable broth
Salt and pepper to taste

Directions:

1. Chop garlic and let sit for 5 minutes to enhance its health-promoting properties.
2. Remove stems from mushrooms and slice the mushroom caps.
3. Heat broth in a stainless steel skillet. When broth begins to steam, add mushrooms and Healthy Sauté, covered, for 3 minutes.
4. Remove skillet cover and let mushrooms cook for 4 more minutes, stirring constantly.
5. Place in a bowl and add garlic, olive oil and salt and pepper while it is still hot.

Serves 1

Nutritional Profile							
Calories	85	Carbohydrates	16.66 g	Saturated Fat	0.04 g	Calcium	10.87 mg
Calories-Saturated Fat	0	Dietary Fiber	5.73 g	Fat - Total	1.26 g	Potassium	720.84 mg
Protein	5.72 g	Soluble Fiber	0 g	Cholesterol	0 mg	Sodium	27.67 mg

Healthy Sautéed Red Cabbage

If you are used to eating green cabbage I encourage you to try the special flavor and nutrients found in red cabbage. It tastes great and is rich in vitamins A, C and K.

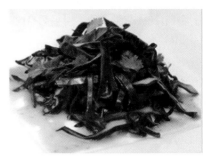

Ingredients:

1 medium clove garlic, chopped
5 TBS low-sodium vegetable or chicken broth
½ small head red cabbage, shredded
½ TBS lemon juice
¼ TBS extra virgin olive oil
Salt and pepper to taste
Optional ingredient: 1 TBS grated ginger

Directions:

1.   Chop garlic and let it sit for 5 minutes to bring out its health-promoting properties.
2.   Heat 5 TBS of broth in a large skillet. When broth begins to steam, add cabbage, sprinkle with 1 teaspoon lemon juice, cover and cook for 5 minutes.
3.   Transfer to a bowl. For more flavor, cut cabbage into small pieces and toss with garlic and the remaining ingredients while it is still hot.

Serves 1

Nutritional Profile							
Calories	128	Carbohydrates	22.50 g	Saturated Fat	0.63 g	Calcium	132.32 mg
Calories-Saturated Fat	6	Dietary Fiber	6.02 g	Fat - Total	4.19 g	Potassium	736.63 mg
Protein	4.93 g	Soluble Fiber	0.30 g	Cholesterol	0 mg	Sodium	88.13 mg

Mediterranean Hummus

This Middle Eastern dish adds a great appetizer or snack to your *Calorie-Lowering* menu. Rich in protein and dietary fiber, it helps curb your hunger and keeps you feeling satisfied between meals.

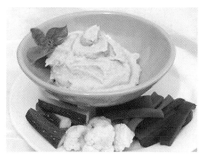

Ingredients:

2 cups cooked garbanzo beans (or 1-15 oz can (no BPA))
2 TBS low-sodium chicken broth
1 TBS + 2 TBS extra virgin olive oil
2 cloves medium garlic, chopped
1 TBS tahini (sesame butter)
1 TBS lemon juice
Salt and pepper to taste

Directions:

1.   Blend garbanzo beans, chicken broth, 1 TBS extra virgin olive oil, garlic, tahini, and lemon juice in blender or food processor. Add the 2 TBS olive oil a little at a time through the feed hole as the mixture is blending.

2.   Season to taste with salt and pepper.
       Serve each serving of hummus with crudités.

Serves 6

Nutritional Profile							
Calories	167	Carbohydrates	16.14 g	Saturated Fat	1.34 g	Calcium	32.50 mg
Calories Saturated Fat	12.08	Dietary Fiber	4.30 g	Fat - Total	9.78 g	Potassium	182.02 mg
Protein	5.45 g	Soluble Fiber	1.29 g	Cholesterol	0 mg	Sodium	6.40 mg

Recipes
Desserts

10-Minute Fresh Berry Dessert with Yogurt and Chocolate

Weight Loss Success is not about deprivation, so this tasty dessert is a great way to treat yourself—and it's nutritious too!

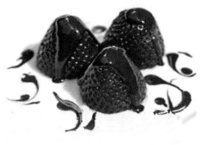

Ingredients:

½ - 8-oz basket fresh strawberries or raspberries
4 oz nonfat vanilla yogurt
1 oz-wt dark chocolate

Directions:

1. Fold together berries and yogurt.
2. Melt chocolate in a double boiler with heat on medium. Place berries and yogurt in a bowl and drizzle with melted chocolate.
3. For a more formal presentation you may want to pour a pool of yogurt on a plate and place berries on top of pool. Drizzle chocolate over berries as shown in photo.

Serves 1

Nutritional Profile							
Calories	291	Carbohydrates	46.20 g	Saturated Fat	6.61 g	Calcium	231.71 mg
Calories-Saturated Fat	59	Dietary Fiber	9.26 g	Fat - Total	9.71 g	Potassium	419.57 mg
Protein	8.84 g	Soluble Fiber	0 g	Cholesterol	5.67 mg	Sodium	134.57 mg

5-Minute Ginger Pineapple

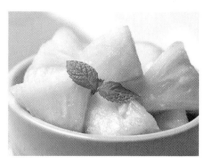

Fruit is a great way to satisfy your sweet tooth without adding many calories to your *Calorie-Lowering Plan*. The ginger adds a zing to this recipe, which is an rich source of vitamin C and manganese.

Ingredients:

¼ medium pineapple
½ tsp finely minced fresh ginger

Directions:

1.   Cut pineapple into 1-inch chunks.
2.   Combine pineapple and minced ginger in a bowl and refrigerate for ½ hour.

Serves 1

Healthy Cooking Tips:

Best eaten within an hour.

Nutritional Profile							
Calories	114	Carbohydrates	29.86 g	Saturated Fat	0.02 g	Calcium	29.57 mg
Calories-Saturated Fat	0.20	Dietary Fiber	3.19 g	Fat - Total	0.28 g	Potassium	250.76 mg
Protein	1.24 g	Soluble Fiber	-- g	Cholesterol	0 mg	Sodium	2.39 mg

10-Minute Orange Treat

This easy-to-prepare dessert is a great example of how a dessert can be flavorful and nutritious. Enjoy its tangy flavor and rich source of fiber and vitamins

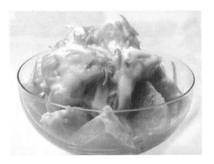

Ingredients:

¼ tsp grated lemon rind*
¼ TBS fresh lemon juice
1 TBS honey
1-¼ TBS nonfat yogurt
1 medium orange
Optional: Top with orange zest

Directions:

1. In a small bowl, whisk lemon rind, lemon juice and honey until the honey is incorporated.
2. Add yogurt and whisk thoroughly.
3. Peel and separate the individual sections of the orange. Be sure to remove the membrane covering from each section. Cut the sections into thirds crosswise. Place in 2 dessert bowls.
4. Spoon sauce over the oranges.

*Use an organic lemon for zest, if possible.

Serves 1

Nutritional Profile							
Calories	143	Carbohydrates	35.67 g	Saturated Fat	0.17 g	Calcium	86.66 mg
Calories-Saturated Fat	2	Dietary Fiber	3.20 g	Fat - Total	0.40 g	Potassium	294.68 mg
Protein	2.25 g	Soluble Fiber	2.07 g	Cholesterol	0.96 mg	Sodium	13.51 mg

SECTION 3

Why Nutrient-Rich World's Healthiest Foods Are Important to Weight Loss Success

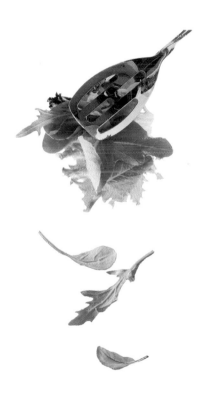

CHAPTER 10

World's Healthiest Foods Reduce Inflammation

In this chapter I want to share with you a new area of health research: the role of inflammation on healthy weight loss. Although my special focus is going to be on inflammation, I will also be telling you about your fat-burning processes, and the best way for you to avoid certain problems in these areas.

What is Inflammation?

We hear a lot about inflammation these days and how it contributes to health conditions such as cardiovascular disease and arthritis. Before I discuss the link between inflammation and weight management, I wanted to first explain what inflammation is.

Inflammation is actually a natural biological response that occurs in the body. Inflammation, in general, is not bad and we don't want to stop the entirety of inflammatory mechanisms in our body if we want to promote good health. What we want to do is control inflammation and not have excess inflammation occurring in our body. It is imbalanced inflammation that can propagate health conditions and related symptoms.

Reducing Fat Storage Cells and Controlling Inflammation

The study of fat cells and their role in health has produced some great surprises in the past 10 years, including the knowledge that fat cells are anything but inactive storage spots for fat. We are used to thinking of our body fat as "just sitting there," placing extra weight on our bones, and stressing our heart and joints from the sheer extra poundage.

What we have learned in the past 10 years is that fat cells are metabolically active, and when too much fat is stored up inside them, they go to work sending off messages that act to increase inflammation and inflammatory problems. Some of the messaging molecules that signal inflammation are only produced in overly fatty fat cells! Conversely, fat cells are also capable of producing anti-inflammatory molecules, and production of these molecules can be reduced when the fat cells become overloaded with fat.

You may already have heard about a weight loss program called *The Fat Resistance Diet* by Dr. Leo Galland (Broadway Books, 2005) or a second weight loss approach called *UltraMetabolism: The Simple Plan for Automatic Weight Loss* by Dr. Mark Hyman (Scribner, 2006). Both of these programs recognize several newly found connections between weight management, our brains, our fat cells, and inflammation. There are a good number of important and cutting-edge facts that you are going to want to consider in your healthy weight loss planning when it comes to inflammation. For this reason, I am going to tell you about this inflammation story in a more detailed way.

Understanding Fat Cells and Leptin

Leptin is a particularly important molecule that our fat cells produce. When we have too little fat stored up inside our fat cells, our fat cells cut way back on their production of leptin.

The reverse set of events holds true when we overeat and our fat stores become too great. Under those conditions, our fat cells start to produce more and more leptin. The increased production of

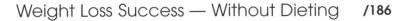

leptin in turn will trigger two sets of events: it will decrease our appetite and it will increase our body's ability to burn fat.

At this point in the story, we have come to the role of inflammation. It turns out that most people who have too much fat stored up in their fat cells also have plenty of leptin. Their fat cells seem to do a good job when it comes to increasing production of leptin when this molecule is needed to help lower appetite and increase fat burning. However, despite having this plentiful supply of leptin, the leptin does not seem to do its job effectively. The appetite reduction and increased fat burn do not seem to take place, even though there is more leptin being produced. This clearly problematic situation is called leptin resistance. Our bodies seem to resist the effects of leptin, even though they would definitely benefit if leptin could do its job.

Research studies make it clear that inflammation is one factor that can contribute to leptin resistance. In fact, it may be the major factor involved with leptin resistance for many individuals. Although it is not yet clear exactly how the two are connected, individuals with chronic, low-grade inflammation are at greater risk for leptin resistance. Anyone living or eating in a way that increases their risk of chronic, unwanted inflammation is also increasing their risk of appetite problems and fat-burning problems due to this problem of leptin resistance. This set of facts is one clear reason to why a Healthiest Way of Eating includes a significant amount of foods that have anti-inflammatory properties.

Adiponectin Can Also Impact Weight Loss

Like leptin, adiponectin is a regulatory molecule produced by our fat cells. Unlike leptin, however, adiponectin will be produced in lower supplies (not greater supplies) by our fat cells when we overeat and start storing up too much unwanted body fat. Adiponectin acts somewhat like a "fat protector," making sure that enough fat will be around in times of short energy supplies. However, excessive and continual overeating that results in chronic deficiency of adiponectin is harmful, not helpful, to our health.

Adiponectin is one of the anti-inflammatory fat-cell-produced molecules that suffers when fat cells become overly loaded with fat. And when the production of adiponectin drops, the body's ability to balance blood sugar also drops. The reason is simple. Adiponectin produced by fat cells is a protein that helps insulin bind onto cells and encourages the flow of sugar out of the bloodstream and into the cells. When fat cells stop producing enough adiponectin, too much sugar stays in the blood

Keeping Inflammation in Check

What does this complicated set of events mean for a meal plan based on the *World's Healthiest Foods*? First, it means that a diet that can prevent over-accumulation of fat in fat cells is highly desirable. What diet best prevents over-accumulation of fat in fat cells? Research suggests it is the diet that contains the greatest percentage of nutrient-rich foods such as the *World's Healthiest Foods*—foods that provide the best variety and quantity of nutrients for the least amount of calories. Second, it means that blood sugar balance and inflammatory balance are extremely important when weight is a problem. Because the *World's Healthiest Foods* are concentrated in nutrients required for blood sugar regulation, insulin regulation, and inflammatory balance, they are also some of your best bets to include in your diet when you have excess fat in your fat cells. They are the perfect foods for getting you safely from here (excess fat in fat cells) to there (fat cells not triggering inflammation from excess storage of fat).

I believe that avoidance of chronic inflammation plays a very important role in weight management. If the body is experiencing too much inflammation, it will not only risk damage to cells and tissues—and cause a domino-like cascade that can lead to disease—but it will also tax our nutrient supplies. It will beckon for antioxidant and anti-inflammatory nutrients to help stave off untoward physiological events. This process will in turn reduce the supply of nutrients that our body has available to accomplish its other functions.

Remember also that inflammation can upset the metabolism that is going on in our fat cells and disrupt the communication that our fats cells are trying to have with our brain, digestive system, and blood-stream. By disrupting our fat cell metabolism, inflammation can confront us with a new risk related to food. This risk is unrelated to any temptations that we might feel. It's a risk of overeating that stems from disruption in the control of our appetite and control of our fat burning processes.

Whether you are trying to lose weight, maintain a recent weight loss, or healthfully maintain the ideal weight you have been at for a while, it pays to stay well nourished in a way that allows your metabolism to adjust along with your new or changing weight. You will be short-changing your metabolism if you drain too many nutrient resources while trying to cope with chronic inflammation.

The last few years of research about inflammation and obesity make me more convinced than ever about the value of the *World's Healthiest Foods*! I have always believed that nutrient-richness was a key to successful weight loss. How could a person possibly go through a challenging period of time like weight loss without needing more nutritional support for their body's metabolism? The answer is: they couldn't! But how could a person get more nutritional support at a time when they clearly needed to eat less food? The answer nutrient-richness—pack more nourishment in fewer calories.

Now research studies have given us the added issue of inflammation. They have told us that inflammation is the part of obesity that can lead to diabetes and heart disease. Inflammation is the part of obesity that can even lead to premature death. This new set of discoveries about inflammation has made us realize what's really at stake when we are trying to lose weight. When we undertake the weight loss process, we are not only trying to lower some numbers on the scale or fit back into old clothes. We are also trying to prevent our bodies from becoming metabolically out-of-balance in a potentially permanent way that will go far beyond the presence of unwanted fat around our middle.

The obesity-inflammation research has made me realize how important the nutrient-rich anti-inflammatory diet—an approach to eating that will prevent the occurrence of unwanted inflammation and avoid that slippery slope between obesity and diabetes and heart disease—really is. But what's most exciting for me to report is the ability of the *World's Healthiest Foods* to accomplish both tasks at once. The same foods that provide you with the highest forms of nutrient-richness simultaneously provide you with the very best anti-inflammatory nutrients. These nutrients include omega-3 fatty acids, many vitamins and minerals, flavonoids, carotenoids, and a long list of other phytonutrients that are unsurpassed in other foods. Read on to learn more about these health-promoting nutrients.

Food Choices Can Help Prevent Inflammation

Always keep in mind that what you eat can help with inflammation in three different ways. These three aspects are taken into consideration in the *Calorie-Lowering Plan* which will show you examples of how to construct a nutrient-rich way of eating that helps to keep inflammation in check.

First, what you eat can be adjusted to avoid deficiency of anti-inflammatory nutrients. An inadequate supply of omega-3 fatty acids, for example, can increase the risk of chronic inflammation. By adjusting the diet to include more omega-3s, the risk of chronic inflammation can be lowered.

Second, what you eat can be adjusted to avoid triggering too much inflammation. Since toxins found in food can serve as inflammatory triggers, you can lower your risk of unwanted and chronic inflammation by eliminating these toxins from your meal plan as much as possible.

Finally, a diet can be adjusted to avoid imbalances that trigger chronic inflammation. A diet that contains too many processed foods, for example, will provide too many calories in the form of simple sugars and too few calories from nutrient-rich foods. By shifting the balance in this area, unwanted inflammation can become less likely. Let's look at some basic dos and don'ts in each of these three areas.

Getting Plenty of Anti-Inflammatory Nutrients

At the top of the list for anti-inflammatory nutrients are two broad groups of phytonutrients called flavonoids and carotenoids. Many flavonoids and carotenoids have strong anti-inflammatory properties, which are often unique to the specific food involved. Richly colored vegetables and fruits are some of your best bets here, including dark green leafy vegetables, beets, and berries. Pineapple also contains a proteolytic (protein-digesting) enzyme called bromelain that has been shown to have anti-inflammatory activity. These foods are included among the *World's Healthiest Foods*.

Some research studies have found that some individuals with high intake of flavonoids and carotenoids do not show reduced tendency to chronic inflammation. These studies make it clear that there are no "magic bullets" when it comes to dietary prevention of chronic disease. While it's important to ensure that you are getting adequate supplies of carotenoids and flavonoids, this shouldn't be at the expense of other nutrients, since all are important. Yet, luckily since carotenoid- and flavonoid-containing foods are also generally rich in so many other vitamins and minerals, they can make great overall contributions to your nutrient goals.

Foods rich in omega-3 fatty acids can also be considered anti-inflammatory because omega-3 fatty acids like alpha-linolenic acid (ALA), eicosapentaenoic acid (EPA), and docosahexaenoic acid (DHA) can be converted into regulatory molecules that put the brakes on inflammation. Foods rich in omega-3 fatty acids include: fish such as salmon, sardines, tuna, and other cold-water fish; and, nuts and seeds, especially flaxseeds, hemp seeds, and walnuts. Other foods that contain omega-3s in lesser, but still very helpful, amounts include soybeans, winter squash, and purslane.

Extra virgin olive oil is another food that has been shown to have anti-inflammatory benefits. Some of these benefits come from oleuropein and hydroxytyrosol, two unique polyphenols found in olives. It is important to note that these two phytonutrients are more concentrated in extra virgin olive than in other types of olive oil. As you'll see in the *Calorie-Lowering Plan,* I place a strong emphasis on extra virgin olive oil because it has such great health benefits.

Avoiding Inflammatory Triggers in Your Meal Plan

Artificial additives, including colors, flavors, and preservatives can all trigger unwanted inflammatory response in the body, not only in the digestive system, but in other body systems once these food toxins get absorbed. On a day-in and day-out basis, processed foods containing these additives can trigger chronic, low-level inflammation throughout the body. The *Calorie-Lowering Plan* avoid these inflammatory triggers.

To lower your risk in this area, your best bet is to choose whole foods that are organically grown whenever possible. Locally grown, seasonal foods are also usually lower in total toxins because they have undergone processing and don't require the same kind of preservation for extended shelf life. If you cannot purchase either organic or seasonal, locally grown foods, fresh whole foods—like fresh fruits and vegetables in their whole, natural form—are still likely to be lower in total toxins than processed foods found in pre-packaged frozen dinners or other pre-packaged items.

Achieving a Dietary Balance That Will Prevent Unwanted Inflammation

Overall dietary balance (and lifestyle balance as well) is extremely important in preventing chronic inflammation. It's impossible for any nutrient, or even a large group of nutrients, to overcome the problems associated with an unbalanced diet. If your diet includes too much fat (especially long chain saturated fat), too many processed foods with simple sugars and little fiber, inadequate protein, too many calories, too few calories, poor timing, or poor eating habits (like inadequate chewing and eating under stress), it is going to be impossible for your anti-inflammatory nutrients to do their job.

This same word of caution applies to lifestyle. Multiple studies show the powerful role of regular exercise in reducing risk of chronic inflammation. Healthy and adequate sleep is also clearly documented as an important component of an anti-inflammatory lifestyle. Don't count on your diet alone to offset a long list of imbalanced living habits. But given a chance within the context of reasonable life choices, an approach to eating—such as that outlined in the *Healthy Weight Loss Eating Plan*—can take you a long way down the path of reduced inflammatory risk.

Achieving an Anti-Inflammatory Dietary Balance

I want you to know that the inflammation story is by no means complete, and you can expect to see plenty of new research in this area, including research related to weight loss. Some of the most fascinating research might come in the area of cells and their development.

Already, many scientists believe that some of our cells actually pass through a kind of decision point, in which they have to decide whether to become fat cells, or whether to become another type of cell, called macrophages. Macrophages are cells that come from white blood cells and form a very important part of our body's immune system. Their name in Greek comes from *makros* meaning "big" and *phagein* meaning "eat." As "big eaters," macrophages are designed to help our body get rid of dangerous substances and micro-organisms that might pose a threat to our health.

In some individuals, nearly half of the cells found in fat tissue (adipose tissue) might be made up of macrophages. This very close connection between our fat cells and our immune system is likely to give us a new understanding of the events involved with excess fat storage and also with loss of stored fat.

Beyond the inflammation question is also the general recognition that weight loss is not simply a matter of counting calories. It's also a matter of our physiological health, metabolic regulation of our appetite, our fat burning processes, and other aspects of our metabolism. I do not expect future research to ever "let us off the hook" when it comes to calories or temptations or other all-too-familiar aspects of weight loss. But I do expect it to add new factors into the mix and to give us new and unexpected ways to succeed in this aspect of our health!

CHAPTER 11

World's Healthiest Foods Balance Blood Sugar Levels

Keeping Blood Sugar Balanced

Glucose—a type of sugar found in our blood—is a necessary nutrient for many cells, especially the brain. An essential feature of maintaining health is to have balanced blood glucose levels. If these levels are too low, our cells may not be properly nourished. If these levels are too high, metabolic consequences can occur which can lead to damage to the kidneys, arteries, and other body systems. High blood glucose levels also usually reflect that the cells are not being able to take in the glucose and therefore are not getting the energy they need for normal function.

When we speak about blood sugar, we are not talking about the same type of sugar as table sugar. Blood sugar is glucose, a simple sugar that others can be broken down into.

At every moment of every day, our blood sugar level is shifting slightly. Eating a meal can shift our blood sugar level dramatically— depending, of course, on which foods we eat and how thoroughly we are able to chew and digest them. It's natural for our blood sugar to increase after a meal. However, it's unnatural for it to increase beyond certain limits. Similarly, between meals, it is natural for our blood sugar to drop. But excessive drops are problematic.

If we eat in a way that turns our blood sugar balance into a roller-coaster ride, we risk several unwanted consequences, including the possibility of unwanted weight gain. The connection between large blood sugar swings and potential weight gain is fairly simple. If our blood sugar goes up too dramatically and then drops, we may experience this drop-off as a need for more food to raise our blood sugar back up again, often to its elevated level. Similarly, if we go too long without eating and our blood sugar "bottoms out" at an excessively low level, we may feel desperate for whatever we can get our hands on. In either direction, the rollercoaster ride can spell trouble for excess eating.

If we get caught up in large pendulum swings with our blood sugar, we are more likely to want high-sugar, high-calorie, and nutrient-poor foods. That situation can only increase our risk of unwanted weight gain.

Processed foods with high levels of simple sugar will spike our blood sugar up more quickly than whole, natural foods. These processed foods are often storehouses of refined carbohydrates, almost never contain enough fiber to balance digestion and provide for a very gradual breakdown and release of carbohydrates into our digestive tract, and are usually deficient in the vitamins and minerals needed to support insulin production and the uptake of glucose into our cells. This can trigger a yo-yo effect in our blood sugar levels and also increase our risk of unwanted weight gain.

Nutrient-rich *World's Healthiest Foods* contain a wealth of vitamins, minerals, fiber, and other health-promoting compounds that can help us maintain optimal blood sugar regulation. They are rich in fiber, which steadies the speed of digestion. They contain chromium and vitamin B3, which are involved in the process of insulin metabolism and the ability of this hormone to clear sugar from our bloodstream. Many nutrient-rich *World's Healthiest Foods* are also storehouses of zinc, a mineral that plays an important role in blood sugar balance.

So, you can see how eating nutrient-rich *World's Healthiest Foods* can help to keep your blood sugar on par. Not only will this nutrient contribution help with your ability to lose weight but it will also provide you with great overall health benefits since excess blood sugar levels can lead to insulin resistance, a condition that we now recognize as a critical factor in the development of many health conditions.

Insulin Resistance

Health scientists have always looked at the process of developing a chronic disease—like obesity, or diabetes, or high blood pressure—as being a complicated one that involves many factors. One of the most prominent factors in this mix is insulin resistance. In the year 2007 alone, over 900 research studies focused exclusively on insulin resistance and its relationship to long-term health. Insulin resistance has become so important in our understanding of health that it is no longer possible to understand a simple process like chronic weight gain without considering insulin resistance and its potential role in the process.

How Insulin Resistance Becomes a Problem

The most common source of energy in our body is sugar (glucose) When our cells need energy, sugar is the fuel they depend on most often. The sugar needed by our cells is constantly flowing through our blood. However, the help of insulin—a protein hormone made by our pancreas—is usually required in order for sugar to leave our bloodstream and flow into our cells. Insulin resistance is a situation in which this process breaks down and our cells stop responding effectively to the insulin produced by our pancreas. Our pancreas may make an unusually high amount of insulin in an effort to get sugar into our cells. But insulin resistance prevents this effort from being fully effective because the actions of insulin continue to be resisted in some way. "Insulin resistance" is the name given to this unwanted set of events. Insulin resistance can become more than just temporary— it can become an everyday roadblock to health.

How Insulin Resistance Affects Weight Management

There is not one simple, easy-to-describe relationship between insulin resistance and body weight. But there are several easy-to-describe features. First, excess body weight in the form of excess fat—particularly around the middle (or abdomen)—is closely related to development of insulin resistance. Particularly when a man has a waist circumference of more than 40 inches or a woman's is 35 inches or more, insulin resistance is significantly more likely to occur.

How does excess abdominal fat help to trigger insulin resistance? Researchers are not entirely certain about this set of events. Traditionally, all of the research on insulin and blood sugar balance has focused on muscle rather than fat. When insulin helps sugar leave the bloodstream, it usually helps sugar enter a muscle cell—not a fat cell.

Until recently, the role of fat cells in blood sugar balance has been overlooked because the muscles have been viewed as so very important in receiving sugar from the blood. Current research, however, has made it clear that fat cells (called adipose tissue) also play a key role in insulin metabolism and blood sugar regulation. One of these connections, as described in the chapter on inflammation, is related to the fact that overly fatty fat cells start making insufficient amounts of adiponectin, a protein that helps insulin to lock onto cells and escort sugar out of our blood. When adiponectin is in short supply, too much sugar can remain in the blood, causing our pancreas to produce more insulin in an effort to compensate. But the true problem cannot be solved by more insulin. The true problem is insulin resistance—in this case, being caused by too much abdominal body fat.

Insulin Resistance and the Tendency to Become Overweight

Just as too much abdominal fat can increase our tendency to develop insulin resistance, insulin resistance can increase our tendency to become overweight. Particularly in women who are lean and have lower amounts of total body fat, insulin resistance increases the chance of weight gain and obesity. Women who have gone through menopause also have increased risk of weight gain following the development of insulin resistance. In women who are already obese, however, insulin resistance may actually protect against weight gain and make weight loss easier. Finally, there is some fascinating research showing that individuals who develop insulin resistance— and at the same time obtain a high percent of their total calories from fat—have a greater chance of gaining weight and becoming obese than individuals who have insulin resistance but obtain only a moderate percent of total calories from fat.

How the World's Healthiest Foods Can Help Prevent Insulin Resistance and Unwanted Weight Gain

There are two basic ways in which your diet can help prevent insulin resistance. Fortunately, the *World's Healthiest Foods* can help you in each of these two basic ways.

First is the task of avoiding a high-fat diet. People who develop insulin resistance—and at the same time obtain a high percent of their total calories from fat—have a greater chance of gaining weight than people who have insulin resistance but obtain only a moderate percent of total calories from fat. As you'll see, the menus that I provide in the *Calorie-Lowering Plan* provide an average of 412 total calories from fat. This is ideal for moderating fat intake and keeping the risk of weight gain down from an insulin resistance standpoint.

Second, and perhaps most important, is steadying your blood sugar as much as possible by the way you eat. Here the *World's Healthiest Foods* can help you in a variety of ways. High-fiber foods are essential for stabilizing your blood sugar because they help regulate the pace of your digestion. And since most of the *World's Healthiest Foods* are plant-based foods they are naturally rich in fiber.

Also important for stabilizing blood sugar are protein-rich foods. Protein digests at a moderate pace that is easy on blood sugar levels. The lean meats, fish, low-fat dairy foods, legumes, and most of the nuts and seeds included as *World's Healthiest Foods* are considered rich protein sources. Once again, the recipes included in the *Calorie-Lowering Plan* frequently feature these protein-rich foods.

Finally, nothing is harder on our blood sugar levels than a diet filled with highly processed foods in which the fiber, vitamins, and minerals have been largely removed through processing. Since the *Calorie-Lowering Plan* emphasizes *World's Healthiest Foods* it keeps these processed foods out of your mainstream meal plan, and in this way, it pays huge dividends in terms of blood sugar balance.

Maintaining Balanced Blood Sugar Levels by Choosing Foods Based on the Glycemic Index

It's important to remember that not all foods, not even all of the *World's Healthiest Foods*, are created alike when it comes to their effects on our blood sugar. Some foods can cause stark spikes while others keep circulating blood sugar levels on a relatively even keel.

The Glycemic Index (GI) is a numerical scale used to indicate how fast and how high a particular food can raise our blood glucose (blood sugar) level. A food with a low GI will typically prompt a moderate rise in blood glucose, while a food with a high GI may cause our blood glucose level to increase above the optimal level. Selecting foods based on their GI is a great way to control fluctuations in your blood sugar levels.

An awareness of foods' GI can help you control your blood sugar levels, and by doing so, may help you to achieve or maintain a healthy weight, let alone prevent heart disease, improve cholesterol levels, and prevent insulin resistance, type 2 diabetes, and certain cancers. A substantial amount of research suggests a low-GI diet provides these significant health benefits and can be a helpful component of a healthy weight loss approach.

The following chart details the GI of the *World's Healthiest Foods*. Next to each food you will find a classification, which are based upon the Canadian Diabetes Association's ranking of GI and their threshold points. Therefore, in this chart, very low is associated with foods that have a GI of 20 or less, low with a GI of 55 or less, medium with a GI of 56-69, and high with a GI of 70 or greater.

FOOD ITEMS	Glycemic Index
VEGETABLES	
Spinach	Low
Lettuce	Low
Zucchini	Low
Asparagus	Low
Cabbage	Low
Celery	Low
Cucumbers	Low
Dill Pickles	Low
Radishes	Low
Broccoli	Low
Brussels Sprouts	Low
Eggplant	Low
Onions	Low
Tomatoes	Low
Cauliflower	Low
Bell Peppers	Low
Green Peas	Low
Squash	Low
GRAIN ITEMS	
Barley	
Pearled barley, cooked	Low
Barley kernel bread (50% kernels)	Medium

Barley flour bread (80% barley, 20% white wheat flour)	High
Whole meal barley porridge	High
Buckwheat	
Buckwheat bread (50% dehusked buckwheat groats, 50% white flour)	Medium
Buckwheat, cooked	High
Corn	
Corn, yellow	High
Corn tortillas	High
Cornmeal, boiled in salted water 2 minutes	High
Millet	
Millet, boiled	High
Oats	
Oat bran bread (45% oat bran, 50% white wheat flour)	Medium
Oatmeal (thick, dehulled oat flakes)	High
Oat bran cereal	High
Muesli	High
Oatmeal (rolled oats), cooked	High
Oat bread (80% intact oat kernels, 20% white wheat flour)	High
Oatmeal (one-minute oats)	High
Rice	
Wild rice	High
Rice cakes	High
Rice noodles, cooked	High
White, boiled	High
Parboiled rice	High
Rice bread	High
Rye	
Rye, whole kernels, cooked	Low
Rye kernel bread (80% kernels, 20% white wheat flour)	High
Whole meal rye bread	High

WHEAT	
Spaghetti, whole meal	Medium
Whole wheat kernels, cooked	Medium
Spaghetti, white, boiled 10-15 minutes	Medium
Cracked wheat, bulgar, boiled	Medium
Wheat kernel bread (80% intact kernels, 20% white wheat flour)	High
Couscous (from semolina-durham wheat,) boiled	High
Whole wheat bread	High
White flour bread	High
Gluten-free	High
FRUITS	
Grapefruit	Low
Apples, dried	Low
Prunes	Low
Apricots, dried	Low
Apples, raw	Low
Pears	Low
Plums	Low
Strawberries	Medium
Oranges	Medium
Pineapple juice	Medium
Grapes	Medium
Orange juice	High
Bananas	High
Kiwifruit	High
Apricots, raw	High
Papaya	High
Pineapple	High
Figs	High
Raisins	High
Cantaloupe	High
Watermelon	High

STARCHY VEGETABLES	
Beets	Medium
Carrots	Medium
Sweet potatoes	High
Potatoes, baked	High
Potatoes, mashed	High
Potatoes, boiled 15 minutes, cubed, peeled	High
LEGUMES	
Soybeans, cooked	Very low
Lentils, red, cooked	Low
Garbanzo beans, boiled	Low
Kidney beans	Low
Lentils, green, cooked	Low
Split peas, yellow, cooked	Low
Soymilk,	Low
Navy beans, cooked	Low
Pinto beans, cooked	Low
Pinto beans, canned	Medium
DAIRY	
Yogurt, low-fat, plain	Very low
Whole fat milk	Low
Skim milk	Low
Yogurt, low-fat, with fruit	Low

My recommendations for considering the GI values of foods in terms of healthy weight loss are:

- Try whenever possible to make the majority of your foods low-GI on a day-by-day basis.
- Allow yourself healthy foods on a daily basis that are medium-GI. However, do not allow these medium-GI foods to become the majority of foods eaten within the day.
- Limit your consumption of high-GI foods. Treat these foods like a special accompaniment to your plan rather than the foundation.

CHAPTER 12

World's Healthiest Foods Promote Energy Production

We all want extra energy—usually at all times, but especially when we think about losing weight. It's common to experience a depletion of energy when we change our food intake patterns or cut back on our overall caloric intake. At these times, it's more important than ever for our food to give us that extra energy boost.

This is one reason why nutrient-rich *World's Healthiest Foods* are so beneficial—they help you feel energized while shedding pounds. And it's quite simple how it happens: the *World's Healthiest Foods* can help energize you by providing your body with ample amounts of nutrients required by the body's energy production systems.

It's not just that they provide you with enough macronutrients (carbohydrates, protein, fat) that serve as the starting place for the production of energy. They also contain micronutrients (vitamins and minerals) that help to release the energy and then recapture it so it can be stored for later use when and where it's most needed.

Capturing energy from the food you eat takes place in your cells. Some of the most important energy production spots are very small microstructures inside our cells called mitochondria. The energy production process that takes place in our mitochondria is a complicated process. To function properly it involves a variety of enzymes that require many vital health-promoting nutrients—such as vitamins B1, B2, B3, B5, and B6, lipoic acid, coenzyme Q, as well as iron, magnesium, and sulfur. So, imagine the difference in how much energy you'll feel from eating nutrient-poor refined foods as opposed to nutrient-rich whole foods such as fresh fruits, salads, and vegetables. These and other *World's Healthiest Foods* will definitely keep your energy systems supplied with the health-promoting nutrients it needs to fuel your vitality.

Additionally, nutrient-rich *World's Healthiest Foods*—especially fruits and vegetables—contain phytonutrients that act as powerful antioxidants. In addition to the many other benefits that these plant-based nutrients provide, they have the ability to support healthy energy production. That's because in the process of making energy, your body also creates oxygen radicals that can damage the mitochondria's energy centers as well as many cells and tissues, leading to reduced and inefficient energy production. But, the phytonutrients and other antioxidants (such as vitamin E) contained in nutrient-rich *World's Healthiest Foods* can act as protective sentries for your cells, quenching oxygen radicals so that they can not do damage.

CHAPTER 13

World's Healthiest Foods Promote Optimal Metabolism

Healthy weight loss involves the burning of body fat, while preserving other tissue (such as muscle mass). While "fat burning" may sound like a fairly simple process, it is anything but.

In chemical terms, "fat burning" means oxidation of fat. In order to breakdown body fat and turn it into energy, many different enzymes and nutrients are required. Directly involved in this process are the vitamins B2 (riboflavin), B3 (niacin), and B5 (pantothenic acid). Also involved are proteins, together with sulfur- and phosphorus-containing molecules. If our food fails to provide us with an ample supply of these fat-metabolizing nutrients, we are not going to burn body fat in an optimal way. That's why it's so important to focus on nutrient-rich *World's Healthiest Foods*—for their concentration of these and other nutrients—when looking to optimize healthy weight loss.

There is also some preliminary research on the role of certain nutrients to induce "thermogenesis" in brown fat cells. The *World's Healthiest Foods*—notably those that provide higher protein and lower refined carbohydrates, as well as those rich in fiber—are integral to activating the thermogenic production of heat in brown adipose (fat) cells. In addition, they decrease storage of dietary fat in ordinary cells; therefore, they may be helpful aspects to consider in the process of weight loss or any aspect of weight management.

I'd like to point out one further area of research involving optimal metabolism and weight loss—that area is contamination of whole, natural foods with pesticides and other toxic substances when these foods are grown and processed in an unhealthy way. There's some preliminary evidence to suggest that chlorine-containing pesticides and other compounds (collectively referred to as "organochlorines") can interrupt the process of thermogenesis and make weight loss more difficult through this means. My emphasis on organically grown foods lets you steer clear of these organochlorine contaminants! You won't have to worry about them potentially interrupting your body's metabolism if you stick as much as possible with organically grown whole foods.

CHAPTER 14

World's Healthiest Foods Help You Manage Adverse Food Reactions

Adverse food reactions (what people may call "food allergies") can cause numerous symptoms and can be the underlying reason for challenges to optimal health. These negative reactions to specific foods are more common than you might expect, and they can be surprisingly difficult to pinpoint as contributing factors to health problems. Adverse food reactions can include food allergies that start in early childhood and continue on throughout life. They can also involve more temporary reactions to food that occur when you are feeling particularly low in energy and when your physical health is especially compromised. But in either case, you will not always have an easy-to-spot symptom that tells you, "Aha! My body is having a problem with something I ate." In the case of adverse food reactions, it's much more likely that you will feel bad in some way (i.e., fatigued, irritable, depressed, foggy headed, lethargic) that could involve dozens of causes. All of the above symptoms, for example, could be caused by lack of sleep, or chronic stress, or a long list of psychological factors.

When we have adverse food reactions, we might be reacting to several different food components. It could be some unique food proteins that are triggering our problematic reactions. It could also be the presence of sugars in food that we lack the enzymes to digest properly. We might also react to food additives and preservatives, or to pesticides or other food contaminants.

Regardless of the food component that is triggering an adverse reaction, you almost always feel better if you can eliminate the food from your meal plan (or at least substantially cut back on your consumption of the food). As you will see later in this chapter, this process of avoiding potentially troublesome foods usually falls under the heading of an "elimination diet." Later in this chapter, I'll be telling you much more about the details of a modified elimination diet that you can follow in your own meal planning as you pursue weight loss and more vibrant health.

Adverse food reactions really boil down to a kind of mismatch between a person and a food. You and I may just not be cut out to eat anything and everything! If you and your food are mismatched, you may have a more difficult time having your body function at an optimal level. Recent reviews of popular weight loss diets clearly show that unusual diets—mismatched not only to a person's nutrient needs but also to a person's broader metabolic pattern—are unsupportive of weight loss in comparison to balanced, metabolically matched diets. Although adverse food reactions have not been specifically studied in this regard, they are established as real-life responses to food that can upset many different metabolic balances in a person's body, and can compromise function in several different body systems, including the digestive system, immune system, nervous system, endocrine system, and inflammatory system. If these body systems are not working well, your path to healthy and optimal weight loss may be compromised.

Two important examples of adverse food reactions—not specifically linked to weight management problems but relatively high up on most research lists of foods most likely to cause adverse reactions— are dairy and wheat. Here's a closer look at each of those foods and their potential for adverse reactions.

In the case of dairy, as many as 15% of all U.S. infants show unwanted reactions to cow's milk, including common symptoms that can be related to many other factors besides food. These symptoms include irritability, fussiness, upset stomach, and bowel problems like excessive gas, bloating, or diarrhea. When tested for food allergy, however, as few as 5% of all infants actually test positive for cow's milk allergy. The frequency of dairy allergy in adults has been estimated in some studies to be similar to the frequency in children, and in other studies to be somewhat lower. (As is the case for all food allergies, we do not have very accurate data to estimate the number of people actually affected.)

In the case of dairy, sometimes the adverse reaction is related to milk sugar (lactose). Not all individuals have enough of the enzyme lactase to break down milk sugar and allow it to digest properly. Unfortunately, in the processed food world, milk sugar (lactose) is often added to non-dairy foods for flavor, and the only way to avoid it is to read the ingredient list on the package. Sliced deli meats, powdered coffee creamers, and ready-to-eat baked goods are examples of foods that can contain lactose. Many individuals also have allergic reactions to special proteins in cow's milk called caseins. Unfortunately, in the processed food world, these proteins are also frequently found in a wide variety of foods in forms like calcium caseinate or sodium caseinate. Hot dogs, deli meats, nutrition bars, and protein powder drinks are examples of foods that can contain casein. Individuals who experience adverse reactions to dairy often feel like their entire dietary balance is affected. The consequences of consuming dairy can detract too much from the satisfaction of eating, or lead to confusion about the trustworthiness of the diet. Under these circumstances, the challenges of weight management often become more difficult.

In the case of wheat, there is even less conclusive research on adverse food reactions than there is for dairy. But scientists continue to investigate links between specific wheat proteins, including gliadin

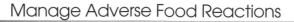

proteins and lectins (especially WGA, or wheat germ agglutinin) and their ability to cause adverse reactions. Much like the situation for lactose and casein in dairy, wheat components find their way into many types of processed foods, and it is possible to experience an adverse reaction to wheat even if you do not eat foods like wheat bread and wheat pasta that are clearly recognizable as wheat-containing foods. The list of processed foods that can contain wheat components includes soy sauce, teriyaki sauce, and seasoning mixes; common processed food ingredients like malt (including barley malt and malt extract) may also contain components of wheat. Like adverse reactions to dairy, adverse reactions to wheat can leave individuals feeling like their entire dietary balance is thrown off, and can increase the difficulty of weight management.

Elimination Diet

I have personally experienced, as well as noticed for others, that adverse food reactions can be a barrier to losing weight. As such, when you embark on your *Weight Loss Success*, if you find that after three weeks of focusing your diet on enjoying the *World's Healthiest Foods* you don't lose any weight, you may want to investigate whether adverse food reactions may be a contributing factor.

What I would recommend in this situation is a modified elimination diet. One of the best tools to use for this is to keep a journal. Write down all the food that you eat at each meal, and then when you reintroduce eliminated foods, write down whether or not you notice experiencing an adverse reaction to them.

I realize that you'll need the help of a licensed healthcare practitioner to diagnose or treat a food allergy, and that you will also need the support of a healthcare practitioner to go on a full-fledged, nutritionally restrictive or nutritionally complicated elimination diet. (I should also point out here that in the case of some full-blown elimination diets, medical monitoring is important from a safety standpoint.) But I am not talking about a full-blown elimination

Cabbage
Carrots
Celery
Collard greens
Garlic
Green beans
Green peas
Kale
Olive oil
Onions
Lettuce
Sea vegetables
Summer squash (zucchini)
Sweet potatoes
Swiss chard
Winter squash
Apples
Grapes
Lemons
Pears

Brown rice

Black beans
Garbonzo beans
Lentils

Pumpkin seeds
Sunflower seeds
Cod
Salmon
Lamb

diet in this situation. I am only talking about some practical steps you can take to experiment with avoidance of foods that are most commonly associated with adverse food reactions. The chart shows the foods that are *less* likely to be associated with these kinds of problematic reactions.

You'll have to decide how comfortable you are restricting your food intake to the above list. If you are worried about staying well-nourished on the above foods, you should consult with a healthcare practitioner rather than attempting these dietary changes on your own. You aren't likely to see many changes in your health or well-being unless you stick with these food modifications for at least one week, so you need to feel comfortable in sticking to this restricted meal plan for that amount of time. At the end of one week, you will want to start re-introducing old foods back into your meal plan. I recommend that you introduce only one food at a time, and that you wait at least two days before re-introducing another food. I would also recommend that you start with aspara-gus, avocados, beets, broccoli, Brussels sprouts, cauliflower, cu-cumbers, blueberries, watermelon, flaxseeds, and quinoa when starting this food re-introduction process since they are not as com-monly associated with adverse food reactions as some of the other foods you might have eliminated from your meal plan.

After that, you will want to continue re-introducing other foods back into your meal plan, on this same one-per-day basis and wait-ing at least two days before you add the next food. While you are re-introducing the foods that you avoided during your week on the modified elimination diet, try to notice any adverse reactions that you may have. Try to pay special attention to any problems that prompted you to experiment with food elimination in the first place. If these problems return, it might be evidence that the newly re-in-troduced food is not well-matched for your body's metabolism and might be worth avoiding in future meal planning.

If you do suspect any adverse reactions using this modified elimina-tion approach, you should definitely consider a consultation with a nutritionist or other healthcare provider who has extensive expe-rience with food allergy. A more structured elimination-challenge diet might also be important to consider. For more information on food allergy and sensitivity, see page 719 of *The World's Healthiest Foods* book.

CHAPTER 15

World's Healthiest Foods Promote Digestive Health

The *World's Healthiest Foods* provide our digestive system with the health-promoting nutrients it needs to function at its best. This is not only important to overall health but to successful weight loss as well.

In order to achieve healthy weight loss, it is necessary to maintain metabolic supplies of energy to our brain, muscles, and other organ systems. This "metabolic maintenance" can only be achieved when the digestive tract is working properly. Your digestive tract is the place where everything starts.

The digestive process begins when you chew your food. It's important to adequately chew in order to break the food down into small enough pieces to allow for the best digestion. I think that the more you chew, the more weight you can lose. Unless you can break down your food effectively, nutrients will not be made available for absorption up into your body. And if you cannot absorb the nutrients, they cannot provide benefits to the rest of your body. It's absolutely essential for you to digest food and absorb nutrients in an optimal way if you want to achieve healthy weight loss.

As I will present in Chapter 10, inflammatory balance in the body may be especially important to maintain during times of weight loss. One way to maintain this balance is to make sure your digestive tract is functioning optimally. That's because if there is any compromise in your digestion, unwanted molecules (like toxic residues or allergy-causing substances) can sometimes get absorbed into the blood stream and trigger unwanted inflammatory responses.

While all nutrients are important to maintaining digestive health, following are a few of the health-promoting nutrients found in the *World's Healthiest Foods* that have been singled out for their special contribution.

Dietary Fiber
At the top of many lists for digestive tract support is dietary fiber. Your food simply cannot pass through you in an optimal way unless it contains fiber. Ideally, we should have at least 10 grams of fiber with every meal and at least 5 grams with every snack, although 20 grams per meal and 10 grams per snack would also be helpful to most of our digestive tracts. Whole, unprocessed foods are essential for adequate fiber. Of special importance are *World's Healthiest Foods* such as vegetables, legumes (like beans or lentils) and whole grains. The skins of fruit are also rich in fiber. Fiber helps keep food moving through our intestines at a gradual pace   not too fast and not too slow.

Glutamine
Although not as well known in the conventional world of nutrition, glutamine is an amino acid that serves as one of the primary fuels for cells that line our small intestine. It can be made from other amino acids found in food or in our body, but it is also found preformed in a variety of *World's Healthiest Foods*, including cabbage, beets, beet, chicken, fish, beans, and dairy products.

Short Chain Fatty Acids
Like glutamine, short chain fatty acids (or SCFAs) are not well-known in the conventional world of nutrition, but these key nutrients serve as preferred fuels for cells that line our large intestine. If these cells do not have adequate energy, they cannot process our food properly. SCFAs are formed by bacteria in our small intestine when these bacteria process starches (especially resistant starches) and several other types of carbohydrate-related molecules found in our food. *World's Healthiest Foods* such as whole grains like corn, oats,

wheat, rye, and brown rice; fruits such as apples and citrus fruits; and all legumes are good sources of resistant starch and non-starch carbohydrates that our intestinal bacteria can convert into SCFAs.

Other Digestive-Health Nutrients

The process of digestion and absorption is a complicated one that involves dozens of different cell types, dozens of different enzymes, the movement of smooth muscles around our intestines, and the trigger of these muscles by our nerves. It's literally impossible to name a single vitamin or mineral that does not play a role either directly or indirectly in some aspect of digestive health. For this reason, foods with the greatest concentration of nutrients and greatest variety of nutrients are optimal for digestive support. The *World's Healthiest Foods* fit this description exactly because they have all been chosen on the basis of nutrient-richness. They provide our digestive tract with all of necessary nutrients, while at the same time avoiding putting pressure on the digestive tract to work unduly hard.

CHAPTER 16

World's Healthiest Foods Promote Liver Health

Dietary balance and nutrient-richness are the keys for supporting your liver and the keys for supporting healthy weight loss as well. Good balance and nutrient-richness work equally well for weight loss and liver health because both processes depend on the same dietary foundation of nourishment.

The *World's Healthiest Foods* are important for delivering a concentrated and varied mixture of metabolic-support nutrients to your liver. If you can choose the certified organic version of nutrient-rich *World's Healthiest Foods* you will also be able to avoid unnecessary metabolic loads on your liver that can occur from toxic residues found in non-organic foods (for more on organic foods, see page 223). Since the *World's Healthiest Foods* are minimally processed foods, they also support liver health by freeing your liver from the task of processing additives. An approach to food that emphasizes the above principles—relying on nutrient-rich *World's Healthiest Foods* as the foundation of your diet, and choosing organically grown varieties when possible—can work wonders for your liver, and in keeping your weight loss process a healthy one.

Why is the liver so important for healthy weight loss? From a metabolic standpoint, losing weight places an extra toll on our body. It's a metabolic challenge for our body to shift from weight maintenance over into weight loss. Alongside of the digestive tract, our liver lies at the very center of this process. Our liver is the place where things get sorted out in terms of metabolism. The breakdown of fat into energy and the transport of unwanted fat both require a healthy liver. So does production of energy to fuel the brain during a time of metabolic stress. Healthy blood sugar balance, healthy wakefulness and sleep, and healthy processing of vitamins and minerals all depend on a healthy liver.

Will you feel healthy enough to stick with your weight loss? Will you be able to sustain the process over many months because you feel healthy and up to the task? The answers to those questions point directly to your liver as the organ system that is focused on metabolic challenges and optimal metabolism. So, as you can see, supporting your liver is a very important aspect of encouraging healthy weight loss and the *World's Healthiest Foods* provide the nutrients that can promote liver health.

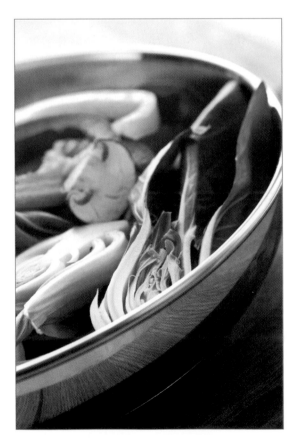

SECTION 4

Weight Loss Success
Q&As

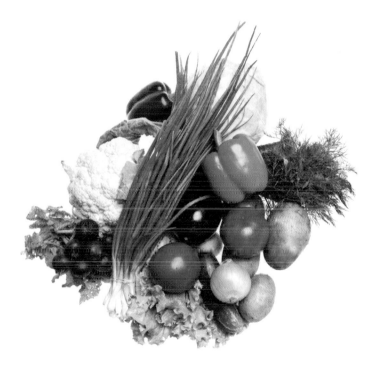

Q&A 1:

What Is a Calorie?

In simplest terms, a calorie isn't any kind of "thing" whatsoever. Calories are not like proteins, or carbohydrates, or vitamins, or any kind of nutrient. You can find protein in food. You can find vitamins in food. Yet, you cannot find a calorie in any food at all. Calories do not exist in that way.

Calories are units of measurement. They are like inches, miles, ounces, degrees of temperature, pounds, tons, gallons, and acres. They are just a way of understanding how much of something is present. In the case of calories, this something is energy. The amount of energy associated with any set of events can be measured in terms of calories. Calories don't have to involve food. For example, there are a specific number of calories that any electrical wire can carry without catching fire. There are a specific number of calories that strike the earth each day in the form of sunlight. Calories are not found in food. They are only related to food insofar as food has the potential to be measured as a form of energy.

Can Food Calories Be Accurately Measured?

Hundreds of Internet website post lists of foods and calories. The U.S. Department of Agriculture publishes a searchable online database (http://www.nal.usda.gov/fnic/foodcomp/search/) with calorie information on thousands of food.

Is the information provided by the USDA and other websites accurate? Unfortunately, the answer is both yes and no. Yes, there are solid scientific studies using real foods and real laboratory conditions to support the specific calorie numbers that appear in the USDA database and in other published lists of food and calories. This research can be very high quality, sophisticated, and scientifically sound. But it is research based on laboratory analysis—not research based on the passage of real food through a person's digestive tract. Unless food gets digested, it cannot provide us with any calories (energy).

When food calories are measured in a lab, a device called a bomb calorimeter is used. This device measures energy in the form of heat. Within this device, a highly oxygenated, sealed chamber containing a food sample is floated in water. An electrical current is used to ignite the food-oxygen mixture, and as it burns, the water surrounding the floating chamber heats up. The number of calories in the food is determined by the change in water temperature. A high-caloric food gets the water hotter by releasing more heat energy than a low-calorie one.

The human body, of course, is not nearly as simple as a lab device. We don't digest food by setting it on fire. We digest chemically, and our biochemistry is highly individual—in fact, unique. The calories of energy we obtain (or don't obtain) from food can vary significantly, and some individuals are better matched to one kind of food versus another. Even though calories can be measured accurately in a lab where they appear to be a fixed attribute of food, once we get inside a living person, and a uniquely biochemical digestive tract, all bets are off when it comes to a rigid set of calorie predictions.

Proteins, Carbohydrates, Fats, and Calories

The laboratory-based rules in nutrition have always been simple: proteins and carbohydrates have traditionally been said to contain 4 calories per gram. Fats have been said to contain 9 calories per gram. This calorie-based description of the three primary macronutrients has been used as the basis for dozens of weight loss programs, especially programs that advocate low-fat, reduced-calorie intake. These programs are based on sound science, but once again, the science is laboratory science, not human digestive tract science.

The reasoning behind these low-fat, calorie-based approaches to weight loss has been simple. Why risk consumption of one macronutrient type (fat) when that nutrient type contains more than twice as many calories (9 per gram) as the other two basic types (protein and carbohydrate at 4 per gram)? While this reasoning seems sound in terms of the mathematics, the successful weight loss experience of many individuals on high-fat, low-carbohydrate diets has seemed to contradict it. But there is not really a contradiction here at all. Individuals are not identical in their digestion. They are differently matched to different foods. Some individuals clearly do better on higher fat, lower carbohydrate diets—even if those diets contain the exact same number of calories as higher carbohydrate, lower fat diets! Figuring out the best dietary balance for your weight management—especially the best balance of proteins, carbohydrates, and fats—is important. It's also a task that is separate from the task of counting calories.

Do Calories Matter?

If human digestion of food is so individualized and different from the laboratory analyses, do the lab analyses of food calories really matter? Yes, they do! No matter how well matched you are to your weight management meal plan, you simply cannot lose weight if you do not pay any attention whatsoever to calorie intake. You cannot lose weight if your body digests food and releases the exact same amount of energy from the food needed to maintain your muscle mass, fat mass, and water weight. In this sense, calories definitely matter. Paying attention to calories is worthwhile. But counting calories isn't the whole story, and it doesn't take the place of health-promoting nutrients that you need to burn fat. The key is that you need more nutrients and fewer calories.

Q&A 2:

Why Are Organic Foods Important to Healthy Weight Loss?

As you know, I am a big proponent of organically grown foods. I believe that they remain your best bet for avoiding food contaminants and optimizing your nutrient intake. But what about weight loss? Are organically grown foods better not only for nourishment, but also for losing or managing weight? While there are no research studies comparing weight loss on an organic food diet versus weight loss while consuming non-organic food, there are bits and pieces of evidence in two areas that have convinced me that it is important to pay increased attention to the benefits of organics when you want to lose weight healthfully.

The first area of evidence involves food contaminants. During periods when we are trying to lose weight, some health risks that would ordinarily not be bothersome can end up posing a significant risk. Toxicity risk from environmental pollutants and food contaminants falls into this category. Research studies have shown that levels of toxins in our bloodstream and tissues can increase during periods of weight loss. In addition, normal metabolic patterns used to detoxify pollutants can become challenged during these periods of time.

The strict rules that apply to production of organic foods dramatically reduce levels of food pollutants, including pesticides, solvents, and heavy metals. These substances can be especially risky when we are following a weight loss diet. During weight loss, we borrow more heavily upon our body stores of nutrients. We use fat in our fat cells for energy—that's one of the primary ways we lose weight (and body fat). But we may also move more minerals in and out of our bones, or more amino acids in and out of our muscles. Even though our body may be getting smaller in dimension and weight during weight loss, the load upon our metabolism can increase greatly. If we've stored up any heavy metals (like lead) in our bones, or fat-soluble toxins (like solvents and some pesticides) in our fat cells, these toxins may be released from their storage spots during weight loss. Our liver and kidneys will be called on to respond to this challenge with more active detoxification—and that challenge in turn will call for more energy and more nutrients.

Weight loss is a period of time when we need to get the most from the least. Weight loss means that we are giving ourselves less food, but simultaneously asking our body to do more metabolically. From a nutritional standpoint, we are placing special premium on the food we do choose to eat. In fact, this reduced amount of food has to accomplish more from a nutritional and metabolic standpoint. Once again, organic food is the ticket to success when it comes to getting the most nutrients from the least amount of food.

From a research standpoint, there continues to be debate over the nutritional differences between organic versus non-organic food. Although a research comparison of organic versus non-organic food seems like a fairly straightforward proposition, nutritional differences of this kind are not always that easy to determine. However, given all of the research studies that we have seen over the past 20 years of research, we believe that the overall evidence clearly shows better nutrient composition in organic versus non-organic food. On average, we believe that this difference falls into the range of 10-20% more available nutrients in organically grown food. We can get more nutrients from the calories we spend, or even cut back on our food without losing nutrients. That's critical at a time when we are challenging our body's metabolism.

Even though you may be emphasizing more fresh fruits and vegetables during a time of weight loss, remember that the benefits of organics aren't limited to these food groups. Nuts, seeds, olive oil, legumes, whole grains, lean meats, and low-fat dairy products will all improve the healthiness of your weight loss if they have been organically grown/raised.

Q&A 3:
What Causes Us To Overeat?

Overeating is an extremely common problem that most everyone has faced at some point in their relationship with food. We overeat for an infinite number of different reasons that range from stress to pleasure to prolonged nutrient deficiency. But there are also some common patterns in overeating, and being aware of these patterns can be helpful for taking steps in another direction.

Emotional Overeating

Our moods can definitely contribute to our risk of overeating. Research studies in this area repeatedly show that negative moods result in greater risk of overeating. These negative moods can include fear, sadness, anger, resentment, frustration, and stress. Sometimes a diet can trigger a negative mood all by itself if the daily food plan is too restrictive, or not enjoyable, or lacking in creativity. One of the reasons I have confidence in the weight-lowering ability of the *World's Healthiest Foods* is the enjoyment we get from eating them! With fresh, whole, natural foods and delicious recipes that are simple to prepare, you are likely to lower your risk of a negative mood triggered by diet alone. Of course, for other sources of negative moods—like work problems, or relationship problems, or ongoing stress—it's important to start working out better lifestyle solutions in these areas.

External Overeating

In a nutshell, external overeating means overeating as a result of too much emphasis on food stimuli that are all around you. We live in a culture that surrounds itself with food, not only in gas station food marts and community gatherings but also in television commercials, billboards, and advertising of every kind. The more wrapped up we get in these cues, the more likely we are to overeat.

In research studies of external overeating, the presence of fast foods, convenience foods, and other instantly available pre-packaged foods is linked with the tendency to overeat. The *World's Healthiest Foods*—while very simple to obtain and prepare—are not "instantly available." Enjoying them as the main components of your daily meal plan takes a little bit of effort. This little bit of effort may in fact pay big dividends by limiting your risk of external overeating.

Restriction-Triggered Overeating

The best-researched pattern when it comes to overeating may be the pattern that is referred to as restriction-triggered overeating. In this pattern, there is basically a rebellion that goes on inside of us when we have put too severe limits on the foods we allow ourselves to eat. The more unreasonably we restrict ourselves, the greater our risk of overeating.

In some cases, researchers have speculated that a specific region of our brain, called the ventromedial prefrontal cortex (VmPFC), may be involved in this pattern of restriction-triggered overeating. The VmPFC is partially responsible for our ability to consider long-term consequences when making an immediate decision. Individuals with damage to this region of their brain more often make decisions that focus only on the here and now, without figuring out how to make long-term consequences work to their advantage. Overly restrictive diets may put us in the exact same kind of predicament: we will tend to forget about the long-term aspects of weight loss and life-long health and instead think only about all of the foods we've missing out on in the past 24 hours. The *Calorie-Lowering Plan* not only avoids overly restrictive eating, but actually encourages daily meal plans that feel normal, natural, tasty, and freely chosen.

Overeating Due to Misjudgment

Overeating does not necessarily mean huge portion sizes that look ridiculously large on your plate. It does not necessarily mean second or third helpings either. When it comes to weight management, most people have a difficult time estimating the amount of food they are eating. A fairly small error in judgment can be the difference between weight loss and weight gain. For example, let's say you consume a salad five days each week, and you think you are using one tablespoon of oil and vinegar dressing on the salad when in fact you are using two tablespoons. Over the course of one year, this difference of one tablespoon will add up to 31,200 calories or nine pounds of weight!

Overeating Is Partly Natural

Eating too much of a tasty food is not only common but also natural. It's natural to want more when a food is delicious. If you judge strictly by the response of your taste buds, you've got a good chance of overeating. That's why I always focus on the issue of nutrient-richness when I recommend the *World's Healthiest Foods* as the mainstay of your weight loss plan. In addition to delicious taste, I know that an optimal supply of nutrients is critical for avoidance of overeating. If you are looking for foods that can provide you with a greater variety of nutrients or a greater quantity of nutrients you don't have to look much farther than the *World's Healthiest Foods*.

Q&A 4:

How is the Calorie-Lowering Plan Similar to the Mediterranean Diet?

The *Calorie-Lowering Plan* is the result of my decades of traveling and researching the foods consumed by populations throughout the world. It is an extension of my Healthiest Way of Eating that is specifically geared towards those who are looking to shed extra pounds.

There are many cultures whose diets may afford them good health. Yet, when it comes to an easily adoptable way of eating that features inherently good-for-you foods as well as a reverence for the way that good food can contribute to health and happiness, I feel that there is no better model than the Mediterranean diet.

The Mediterranean diet is a term used to describe the food intake patterns of individuals living in the Mediterranean region (for example, those in the Greek island of Crete as well as Italy, Spain, Portugal, and Southern France). In addition to olive oil, the Mediterranean diet focuses on fresh vegetables, fresh fruits, fish, nuts, seeds, and legumes/beans, food groups at the foundation of the *World's Healthiest Foods* and the *Calorie-Lowering Plan.*

(Before I continue, it's important to point out that the "diet" in "Mediterranean diet" means the routine foodways of a culture, the foods and beverages that they regularly consume. Although the Mediterranean diet—and the *Calorie-Lowering Plan* that it has inspired—can lead to weight loss, the inclusion of the term "diet" doesn't inherently infer restriction of food intake for the purpose of losing weight, the other common meaning of this word.)

Decades ago, when scientists began studying the cultures along the Mediterranean Sea, they found that they had lower rates of disease and longer life spans than many other populations. The scientists deduced that diet was a major contributor to the Mediterranean people's superior health—including lower rates of heart disease and cancer—laying the foundation for further research that has identified other health benefits and helped to pinpoint the contribution of specific foods highlighted in the Mediterranean diet.

While these health benefits are widely touted as the reason to follow a Mediterranean-inspired diet, there is another benefit that is less well known. It turns that that those who follow the Mediterranean diet have less of a chance of becoming obese than those who follow a typical western-style diet. For example, a study published in 2006 in the medical journal *Nutrition* found that those who adhered to a Mediterranean-style diet were 51% less likely to be obese than those whose diet didn't resemble this healthy way of eating. Mediterranean-diet adherents have also been found to have lower levels of systemic inflammation; since inflammation is an outcome of obesity, and reducing inflammation is a very important facet of a healthy approach to weight loss, a Mediterranean-style diet can also be beneficial to healthy weight loss because of its anti-inflammatory benefits

Q&A 5:
What Is The Difference Between Nutrient-Rich and Energy-Rich Foods?

Nutrient-rich foods aren't the same as energy-rich foods although these two terms sound very similar. It's not nutrients per se that give us energy; from the standpoint of nutrition, the term "energy" is actually synonymous with "calories." High-calorie foods can be metabolized in our cells to provide us with a large amount of energy. Low-calorie foods cannot provide us with much energy in terms of calories. They help support our metabolism in an infinite number of ways, but they cannot provide our muscles and organs with the "get up and go" they need to get us through our day.

As in all health-related matters, it's a question of balance here. We need enough energy-rich foods to give us the caloric energy for our "get up and go," and we need enough nutrient-rich foods to support our metabolism while we're on the move.

I can make it easy for you to lock into an optimal mix of energy-rich and nutrient-rich! Actually, I don't have to do much at all, because the world of natural, whole foods has done it for me. The World's Healthiest Foods approach is not only nutrient-rich, but it balances out energy-richness by including energy-rich foods (like nuts and seeds and olive oil) in your regular meal plan, but also watching out for the overall amount included, especially in recipes and stovetop cooking (since I don't recommend cooking with oil).

I don't let energy-richness get out of hand—but I don't forbid myself to use energy-rich foods in any of my recipes or meals. At the same time, I focus heavily on the nutrient-rich foods that are lower energy in terms of calories—most importantly, fresh vegetables. I use these foods generously in my weight loss approach, and they are a key component for balancing out your overall weight loss.

Q&A 6:

Is My Attitude Towards Weight Loss Important?

The aspect of weight loss that many fad diets overlook does not typically involve food selection, but rather, weight loss attitudes and approaches to the experience of weight loss itself. Although weight loss attitudes and weight loss approaches may not seem nearly as important as food selections during weight loss, scientific research tells us otherwise.

Put most simply, weight loss only seems to work when we treat it like part of our everyday lives. Over and over, studies show that when we step out of our lives to lose weight our success is temporary at best. Our weight loss under these circumstances may last for months, but never for years and years.

What does it mean, to "step out of our lives?" On many weight loss diets, it means giving up one of the most natural of human pleasures—the pleasure of eating! It means giving up the delicious tastes and aromas of food, giving up the pleasures of robust, shared meals with family and friends, and giving up our very self-determination with respect to food choices and food portion sizes. Many weight loss diets ask us to temporarily step out of our lives and to turn our lives completely over to a predetermined script not of our making. We are often asked to build our breakfasts, lunches, and dinners around prepackaged foods that we didn't select, cook, or even choose from a list of favorites. By letting someone else make all of these decisions for us, and by stepping out of our normal role as human beings whose everyday lives include the joys of eating, we are told that our chances of losing weight will improve.

Research studies repeatedly show that weight loss works best when we practice self-determination and self-regulation in our every-day food choices, when we enjoy the foods we eat, and when we make healthy lifestyle choices at every step along the way during weight loss.

There is actually one new approach to weight loss called the HAES approach (Health at Every Size) that has evolved to capture some aspects of the attitude described above. In the HAES approach to weight loss, individuals become "health-centered" rather than "weight-centered." Instead of stepping out of their lives to follow some temporary and unfamiliar diet plan, individuals step further into their lives by focusing on long-term lifestyle habits. They also insist on being healthy and living a healthy lifestyle regardless of their body size on any given day. This is resonant with my perspectives related to the *Calorie-Lowering Plan*; it's not a diet but a way of life where you enjoy delicious tasting nutrient-rich foods.

As you can see from all of the examples described above, our weight loss attitudes are just as important as the foods we choose to eat. While making a place for low-calorie, nutrient-rich foods in our weight loss diet, we must also make room for ourselves!

Q&A 7:

What are some of the factors involved in weight gain?

If you are someone who has struggled with weight management, you are very likely to have scratched your head at some point in your life when you gained weight without any apparent rhyme or reason. From a research perspective, the ease with which many people gain weight can be explained by two basic factors: (1) the fact that we're human and (2) energy balance.

Let's take the human part first. In the world of weight loss research, you'll find a long list of scientific terms that have been invented to describe our humanness in managing our weight. Researchers talk about "flexible cognitive restraint," "reduced food disinhibition," and "decreased food cue susceptibility" when analyzing weight loss patterns. But what do these terms really mean? "Flexible cognitive restraint" means that we sometimes stick with our weight loss plan, but other times we do not. When our thinking tells us to avoid a certain food, sometimes we do and sometimes we don't.

According to researchers, we need to be flexible in these situations. "Reduced food disinhibition" means that when we violate our own weight loss rules, we still don't want to go crazy and eat everything in sight. "Decreased food cue susceptibility" means that the mere sight and smell of a food must not always lure us into eating it. All of these terms are ways of describing our human nature—as human beings, we not only take pleasure in our lives (including the pleasure that comes from food) but we also make mistakes and feel overwhelmed in some situations. The research on weight gain says that weight gain is a natural part of our human experience. Sometimes we gain weight easily simply because we are human!

A second factor in easy weight gain is energy balance—or more precisely, the delicate nature of energy balance for many individuals. Every moment of every day, our bodies need energy to keep going. Energy is needed not only to move our muscles, but also to keep us breathing, keep our heart beating, maintain our body temperature, and to allow for many other bodily functions. Each day, we need to consume sufficient energy in the form of food to fuel these bodily functions. For many individuals, however, this energy amount is relatively small and may often fall into the range of 1,500–1,800 calories per day. If an individual requiring 1,500 calories' worth of food consumes 1,500 calories' worth of food, all is well and energy balance is maintained. But if 1,600 calories' worth of food are consumed, energy balance is lost. In this hypothetical example involving the consumption of 100 extra calories per day, not much weight would be gained in a single day, or even over the course of a week. But over the course of an entire year, this daily difference of 100 calories would add up to a 10-pound weight gain. That's a very delicate balance! Especially in the case of processed foods or fried foods, few of us could accurately determine the difference between a 600-calorie meal and a 700-calorie meal.

Physical exercise is also involved in our energy needs, but in slightly different way than you might expect. While it is true that physical exercise directly burns calories and increases our energy needs in this way, it burns surprisingly few calories in the lives of many individuals. Leisurely-paced walking, for example, tends to burn no more than 5 calories per minute for many adults. While that amount is important, it only translates into 100 calories of energy burning per 20 minutes of leisurely walking, or approximately the same amount of calories found in one tablespoon of dry-roasted nuts. In other words, 20 minutes of leisurely walking doesn't buy us very much room for additional food intake (while still maintaining energy balance).

According to energy balance research, what is more important about physical exercise is its role in building and maintaining our muscle mass. Since muscle tissue is a relatively active type of tissue in our body, building our muscle mass tends to increase our energy needs.

When added together, these two weight gain factors—being human and maintaining a delicate energy balance—help explain why weight gain comes so easily to many individuals. Even with some physical activity, many individuals have very little room to work within their allotted calorie intake. This delicate balance is easily upset because all of us are human, get overwhelmed at times, and make very human mistakes.

From a research perspective, the difficulty of weight loss for many individuals is explained by the same two factors that account for ease of weight gain: (1) the fact that we're human and (2) energy balance. Let's go back to the example already discussed of a person whose energy balance allows consumption of only 1,500 calories per day. If that person wants to lose weight, he or she will need to burn up more than 1,500 calories on a daily basis or consume 100 fewer calories each day. (Here we have the weight gain situation in reverse. Instead of gaining 10 pounds per year while consuming 100 extra calories each day, a person is losing 10 pounds per year while consuming 100 fewer calories each day or burning up 100 more calories.)

By burning up 100 extra calories each day, this person could expect to see about 10 pounds of weight loss per year. Ten pounds per year is less than one pound per month. Now imagine following a weight loss diet for 30 days and then stepping on the scale only to find a weight loss of only one pound! And think how particularly troublesome this result would be if you did not like the weight loss diet you were following, or if you felt like your weight loss diet was preventing you from living your everyday life. This is yet another reason why it's important not to think short-term, as we do when we are on a diet. But to undertake a way of eating for our lifetime that is healthful and enjoyable and that can lead to long-term and lasting weight loss.

APPENDIX 1

The World's Healthiest Foods' Quality Rating System Methodology

The World's Healthiest Foods Quality Rating System Methodology

In order to quantify the nutrient richness of each of the World's Healthiest Foods in this book, *The World's Healthiest Foods* book, and the WHFoods.org website, a team of top nutritionists and I designed the World's Healthiest Foods Quality Rating System ("Rating System").

This Rating System qualifies foods as "excellent," "very good" and "good" sources of nutrients, providing you with a simple, yet reliable, way to determine the nutritional attributes of a food. These quality descriptions don't just take a food's nutrient contribution into consideration; rather, they evaluate this nutrient contribution in relationship to the amount of calories a food contains. This way you can evaluate foods in terms of their ability to maximize your intake of important nutrients without having to exceed your individual caloric intake goals.

To help you better understand the categorization of foods as "excellent," "very good" or "good" sources of a particular nutrient, I want to provide you with some background as to how these quality ratings were derived.

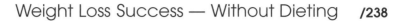

Rating System Categories

We began with a computerized analysis of the nutritional contents of the World's Healthiest Foods using the nutritional analysis software, Food Processor for Windows (ESHA Research, Salem, Oregon, USA). In other words, we started with a food like carrots, and we analyzed how much vitamin C, vitamin A, zinc, protein, etc. that food contained in one commonly eaten serving.

For each food we found the %Daily Value (DV) contribution of each nutrient, as well as the food serving's %DV contribution of calories (for more on DV, see below); the comparison of the two became the Density and is the first (and most important) part of the formula to determine the food's quality rating. We then picked a simple, three-category system for rating all foods: "excellent," "very good," and "good." The definitions of these rating qualifications are as follows:

Excellent	Density>=7.6	And	DV>=10%	Or	DV>=75%
Very Good	Density>=3.4	And	DV>=5%	Or	DV>=50%
Good	Density>=1.5	And	DV>=2.5%	Or	DV>=25%

In reality, the goal that each individual should strive for in terms of daily nutrient and caloric intake varies depending upon his or her personal needs. Yet, to help individuals meet their nutritional needs, government agencies have created standard recommendations for intake. The most up-to-date ones in the U.S. are those created by the Institute of Medicine and are known as the Dietary Reference Intakes (DRIs). Yet, since these DRIs can have many values for each nutrient (varying by age, gender and whether a woman is pregnant or lactating), we chose not to use these as our Daily Value (DV) standard. Rather, for most nutrients we chose to use the U.S. Food and Drug Administration's "Reference Values for

Nutrition Labeling" as our standard for DVs. These are the values used by food manufacturers in the "Food Facts" portion of their product's label.

For other nutrients, such as for those where there were no "Reference Values," we derived a DV based upon the latest research or opinion of nutrition science experts. With respect to omega-3 fatty acids, for example, we adopted the standards set forth in a 1999 workshop conducted at the National Institutes of Health (NIH). The workshop participants—who included prestigious contributors in the field of nutrition science including Artemis Simopoulos, MD, Alexander Leaf, MD, and Norman Salem, Jr., Ph.D—concluded that at least 1.2% of daily calories should come from omega-3 fatty acids, including 1% from alpha-linolenic acid and 0.1% each from EPA (eicosapentaenoic acid) and DHA (docosahexaenoic acid). When translated into the context of an 1800-calorie diet, this workshop standard represented a recommendation of 2.4 grams of omega-3 fatty acids per day, which we adopted as our food and recipe rating system standard, given that we use 1,800 calories as the reference diet for the Rating System. (The 1,800 calories chosen as the reference diet is based upon the Institute of Medicine's recommendation for sedentary women, age 31-50.)

Total Nutrient Richness Chart

Once the density ratings for each food were calculated, I wanted to create a quantitative way that each food's density could be compared. This was the number that was to become the Total Nutrient Richness, featured on page 48. The number is a reflection of how many "excellent," "very good" and "good" ratings a food had. Each "excellent" was assigned a value of 4, each "very good" a value of "2" and each "good" a value of 1. These were added together to arrive at the Total Nutrient Richness score.

APPENDIX 2

Additional Testimonials

Dear Mr. Mateljan,

I have been doing my own research on health and nutrition for almost a year now and I received a copy of your book for Christmas last year. I was very impressed with the wealth of information you provided and your book has become my new bible. Because of you and the research I have done to date, my life has changed tremendously. I am 49 years old and have done a complete change in my lifestyle and I am amazed at the difference it has made in my life. Since I have been following your food guidelines, I have also changed my life in the amount of exercise I do, the amount of water I drink, and I have also learned how to handle my stress better. I have lost weight (not that I really needed to), while I eat more. I have also found more energy and strength. But this is the best part. In 1991, I was diagnosed with Crohns disease after the birth of my daughter. They had me on steroids and taking 21 pills of Asacol for the first year. I am not a pill taker, I despise taking any kind of pills so after the doctor weaned me off the steroids, I stopped taking all pills against his advice. From that point on, I was able to manage my Crohns to some extent and suffered in silence when I would get flare ups. Since I have changed my lifestyle, I have been completely symptom-free for 6 months now. And for that reason, I wish to thank you very much. I also have your 300 Secrets book and I am telling everyone about you and recommending your book. As a matter of fact, I think your book is one of the greatest gifts I could give anyone because it is "the book of life," I look forward to your newsletter and to learning all you have teach me about nutrition (as I am far from being the expert that you are...lol). I am a testament that your knowledge and information shared is priceless. Thank you again. I am one of your biggest fans. — Mitch

PS. I live in Alberta, Canada, and I am enrolling in a University course called "Nutrition 101." I hope someday, I can make a difference in someone's life like you have made a difference in mine. Please keep up the good work and know that your efforts to educate people are not in vain.

I just want to say I've been visiting WHF for a long time. I appreciate the fact that you "get technical" in the descriptions of foods. You don't "dumb it down" but instead explain and go into the science on a molecular level. I have lost 70 pounds (and kept it off) in the last 4 years by changing my exercise/eating habits and the WHFoods List has been a huge help. I have more weight to lose, but by having a scientific understanding of the foods I eat, I'm confident I will reach my goal. — Eleni

A New Life: I just wanted to email to say that your book has truly changed my life. At 22 years old I had just graduated college and was a complete mess; my diet was terrible, I couldn't fall asleep, I was suffering from anxiety, and I weighed 184 pounds which is a lot for someone of my height. My dad borrowed this book from his friend and I started flipping through it and found everything so interesting and appetizing. He quickly purchased it for me and the day I got it I started with the diet plan.

For 4-weeks straight I ate nothing but food from your book and I suddenly felt amazing. I can gladly say that now, with the help of your recipes plus yoga and pilates, that I weigh 145 pounds! Not only did I lose weight but my entire metabolism changed. I no longer had any desire for sweets, or high fat food and the occasional time I do I find that I don't gain weight as quickly. I have lost weight in the past from other diets but always gain it back once I go back to eating badly but this is not a diet, it's a way of life. I swear by your book and make recipes for all my friends and they are picky eaters and love them!

For the first time in my life I feel so happy to just be me... my mood has completely changed, I'm motivated, I have confidence. I feel healthy! Not once do I feel deprived because like I said I don't have cravings anymore! My friends ask me how I do it and I tell them... its all about The World's Healthiest Foods. I feel great and I'm still losing weight! Now I can't wait to get into that bride maid dress! Thank you so much, for changing my life. — Amy

I swapped hamburger for salmon. I ate shrimp instead of bologna. Red grapes make a great substitute for salad dressings.

My thinking became, if you eat anything with enough broccoli or romaine lettuce, it will be okay. Fiber is my friend. All hail green tea.

Cravings for foods I used to eat became virtually nonexistent. My weight loss has been remarkably steady even as I branched out with occasional indulgences. I don't miss anything I used to eat. The World's Healthiest Foods has helped me truly appreciate that I am what I eat." — Mary

I have lost around 24 pounds. I have lots more to go. My husband thinks it will take about another year and one half to lose the rest of my weight. Anyway, your book and website have helped me a bunch. — Sarah

I love and appreciate the site. I have been on a diet since December and lost 45 pounds. The site is incredibly useful in guiding me towards better foods. — Mike

I've read a lot of your stuff and decided to eat more whole grains and eat fruit in between meals. The result was that I didn't get so hungry in between meals and I lost 30 pounds. When my body craves sweets I know what it wants is sugar and then I eat fruit instead. It always helps. — DF

References

Billes, S. K. and Cowley, M. A. Catecholamine Reuptake Inhibition Causes Weight Loss by Increasing Locomotor Activity and Thermogenesis. Neuropsychopharmacology. 2007 Aug 8.

Brand-Miller J. (2005). International GI Database. Human Nutrition Unit, School of Molecular and Microbial Biosciences, University of Sydney, Sydney, Australia. Available online at: www.glycemic index.com.

Buijsse B, Feskens EJM, Schulze MB et al. Fruit and vegetable intakes and subsequent changes in body weight in European populations: results from the project on Diet, Obesity, and Genes (DiO-Genes). Am J Clin Nutr 2009;90(1):202-209.

Cheskin LJ and Kahan S. Low-carbohydrate and Mediterranean diets led to greater weight loss than a low-fat diet in moderately obese adults. Evid. Based Med., Dec 2008; 13: 176.

Cummings, D. E. and Overduin, J. Gastrointestinal regulation of food intake. J Clin Invest. 2007 Jan; 117(1):13-23.

Dhillo, W. S. and Bloom, S. R. Gastrointestinal hormones and regulation of food intake. Horm Metab Res. 2004 Nov 2004 Dec 31; 36(11-12):846-51.

Doucet, E.; St-Pierre, S.; Almeras, N.; Despres, J. P.; Bouchard, C., and Tremblay, A. Evidence for the existence of adaptive thermogenesis during weight loss. Br J Nutr. 2001 Jun; 85(6):715-23.

Epstein LH, Paluch RA, Beecher MD et al. Increasing Healthy Eating vs. Reducing High Energy-dense Foods to Treat Pediatric Obesity. Obesity (2008) 16, 318–326.

Field AE, Haines J, Rosner B et al. Weight-control behaviors and subsequent weight change among adolescents and young adult females. Am J Clin Nutr. 2009 Nov 4. [Epub ahead of print]

Flood A, Mitchell N, Jaeb M et al. Energy density and weight change in a long-term weight-loss trial. Int J Behav Nutr Phys Act. 2009 Aug 14;6:57.

Flood-Obbagy JE and Rolls BJ. The effect of fruit in different forms on energy intake and satiety at a meal. Appetite. 2009 April; 52(2): 416-422. 2009.

Furlow EA and Anderson JW. A systematic review of targeted outcomes associated with a medically supervised commercial weight-loss program. J Am Diet Assoc. 2009 Aug;109(8):1417-21.

Greenberg I, Stampfer MJU, Schwarzfuchs D et al. Adherence and Success in Long-Term Weight Loss Diets: The Dietary Intervention Randomized Controlled Trial (DIRECT). Journal of the American College of Nutrition, Vol. 28, No. 2, 159-168 (2009).

Halton, T. L. and Hu, F. B. The effects of high protein diets on thermogenesis, satiety and weight loss: a critical review. J Am Coll Nutr. 2004 Oct; 23(5):373-85.

Kant AK and Graubard BI. Energy density of diets reported by American adults: association with food group intake, nutrient intake, and body weight. International Journal of Obesity (2005) 29, 950–956.

Kumanyika SK, Wadden TA, Shults J et al. Trial of family and friend support for weight loss in African American adults. Arch Intern Med. 2009 Oct 26;169(19):1795-804.

Larson NI, Neumark-Sztainer D and Story M. Weight Control Behaviors and Dietary Intake among Adolescents and Young Adults: Longitudinal Findings from Project EAT. J Am Diet Assoc. 2009 Nov;109(11):1869-77.

Liu, R.H. Potential synergy of phytochemicals in cancer prevention: mechanism of action. J. Nutr. 2004; 134(12): 34795-85S

Mata J, Silva MN, Vieira PN et al. Motivational "spill-over" during weight control: Increased self-determination and exercise intrinsic motivation predict eating self-regulation. Health Psychol. 2009 Nov;28(6):709-16.

Mendez MA, Popkin BM, Jakszyn P et al. Adherence to a Mediterranean Diet Is Associated with Reduced 3-Year Incidence of Obesity. J. Nutr., Nov 2006; 136: 2934 - 2938.

Mendosa, R. Revised International Table of Glycemic Index (GI) and Glycemic Load (GL) Values - 2002. www.mendosa.com/gilists.htm

Mourao DM, Bressan J, Campbell WW et al. Effects of food form on appetite and energy intake in lean and obese young adults. International Journal of Obesity (2007) 31, 1688–1695.

Newstadt M. Exercise and weight control. J Ky Med Assoc. 2009 Jul;107(7):265-7.

Phelan S, Liu T, Gorin A et al. What Distinguishes Weight-Loss Maintainers from the Treatment-Seeking Obese? Analysis of Environmental, Behavioral, and Psychosocial Variables in Diverse Populations. Ann Behav Med. 2009 Oct 22. [Epub ahead of print]

Provencher V, Bégin C, Tremblay A et al. Health-at-every-size and eating behaviors: 1-year follow-up results of a size acceptance intervention. J Am Diet Assoc. 2009 Nov;109(11):1854-61.

Quatromoni PA, Pencina M, Cobain MR et al. Dietary Quality Predicts Adult Weight Gain: Findings from the Framingham Offspring Study. Obesity (2006) 14, 1383–1391.

Romaguera D, Norat T, Mouw T et al. Adherence to the Mediterranean diet is associated with lower abdominal adiposity in European men and women. J Nutr. 2009 Sep;139(9):1728-37.

Sacks FM, Bray GA, Carey VJ, et al. A weight-loss secret: Calories matter. Comparison of weight-loss diets with different compositions of fat, protein, and carbohydrates. New England Journal of Medicine 2009; 360:859-73.

Savage JS and Birch LL. Patterns of Weight Control Strategies Predict Differences in Women's 4-Year Weight Gain. Obesity (Silver Spring). 2009 Aug 20. [Epub ahead of print]

Savage JS, Marini M, Birch LL et al. Dietary energy density predicts women's weight change over 6 y. The American Journal of Clinical Nutrition. Bethesda: Sep 1, 2008. Vol. 88, Iss. 3; pg 677-684.

Shai I, Schwarzfuchs D, Henkin Y et al. Weight Loss with a Low-Carbohydrate, Mediterranean, or Low-Fat Diet. N. Engl. J. Med., Jul 2008; 359: 229 - 241.

Shixian, Q.; VanCrey, B.; Shi, J.; Kakuda, Y., and Jiang, Y. Green tea extract thermogenesis-induced weight loss by epigallocatechin gallate inhibition of catechol-O-methyltransferase. J Med Food. 2006 Winter; 9(4):451-8.

Tassone, F.; Broglio, F.; Gianotti, L.; Arvat, E.; Ghigo, E., and Maccario, M. Ghrelin and other gastrointestinal peptides involved in the control of food intake. Mini Rev Med Chem. 2007 Jan; 7(1):47-53.

Teixeira PJ, Silva MN, Coutinho SR et al. Mediators of Weight Loss and Weight Loss Maintenance in Middle-aged Women. Obesity (Silver Spring). 2009 Aug 20. [Epub ahead of print]

Tassone, F.; Broglio, F.; Gianotti, L.; Arvat, E.; Ghigo, E., and Maccario, M. Ghrelin and other gastrointestinal peptides involved in the control of food intake. Mini Rev Med Chem. 2007 Jan; 7(1):47-53.

Trichopoulou A, Naska A, Orfanos P, et al. Mediterranean diet in relation to body mass index and waist-to-hip ratio: the Greek European Prospective Investigation into Cancer and Nutrition Study Am. J. Clinical Nutrition, Nov 2005; 82: 935 - 940.

Wang, C. Y., McPherson, K., Marsh. T, et al. Health and economic burden of the projected obesity trends in the USA and the UK. The Lancet, Volume 378, Issue 9793, 27 August-2 September 2011, Pages 815-825

Williams PG, Grafenauer SJ, and O'Shea JE. Cereal grains, legumes, and weight management: a comprehensive review of the scientific evidence. Nutr Rev 2008 Apr; 66(4):171-182.

(INDEX continued on next page)

About the Author

George Mateljan is a best-selling author and world-renowned expert on the Healthiest Way of Eating and Cooking. He is now celebrating ten years of philanthropy and his dedication to help making this a healthier world. His website receives over 1 million visitors per month.

George Mateljan has had a lifelong interest in food. From the time he was five years old, his favorite room in the house was the kitchen, where he watched as his mother lovingly spent hours preparing meals for the family. He still vividly remembers seeing a bowl full of ingredients transformed into dough that rose as if by magic. Then, after the dough went into the oven, he was tantalized by the fragrant aroma of it baking. He loved the wonderful look and taste of golden loaves of warm bread fresh from the oven.

By watching food being prepared for many years, George learned to appreciate the way each season brought forth its own special foods, including fresh fruits and vegetables. In the spring and summer, there were sweet, juicy strawberries, raspberries, apricots, and many types of melons. In the fall, there were apples, oranges, and sweet potatoes. And in the winter, there were hearty root vegetables such as beets, carrots, and potatoes. George's favorite times were the holidays when he helped prepare special festive dishes.

George's continued passion for food sent him to the ends of the earth to learn about it. He has spent over 30 years traveling to over 80 countries around the world. He experienced cuisines from many cultures renowned for their health and longevity and appreciated the different foods and ways of preparing them that were unique to each.

George's education in biochemistry helped his understanding of what he learned through observing, tasting and formal training to create this better and healthier way of cooking. George earned a certificate studying French cuisine at the renowned La Varenne cooking school near Paris. He studied Italian cooking at the Guiliano Bugialli's cooking school in Florence. He refined his skills at the Gourmet's Oxford in England.

George was disappointed that he couldn't find nutritious, tasty, and convenient foods for himself and his family, so in 1970 he founded Health Valley Foods, the first company in the United States to offer healthful prepared foods. As time went on, Health Valley produced thousands of convenient, enjoyable products that were packed with nutrition and flavor yet completely free of the white flour, refined sugar, hydrogenated fats, excess salt, chemical preservatives, and artificial colors that are standard in highly processed foods.

In 1996, George sold Health Valley Foods. He felt that after 26 years he had inspired a number of others to establish companies to produce nutritious, conveniently prepared foods, and it was time to turn his energies and resources toward the next phase of helping people enjoy eating healthier. Today, he shares, free of charge, his passion to help others, and his experiences and knowledge with everyone who wants to know about the "Healthiest Way of Eating" through the not-for-profit George Mateljan Foundation.

Over the years, George had come to identify which foods were among the World's Healthiest. And he also knew that in order to eat them on a regular basis the preparation of these foods had to fit the individual tastes and lifestyles of people in today's busy world. So, George worked to create and develop preparation methods and recipes that allow people to enjoy delicious and exciting flavors in easy and affordable ways. His Foundation supports an extensive website and the publication of books to share this information with you.

George has published five books that have been read and used by Millions of people. This includes his latest book, *The World's Healthiest Foods: Essential Guide for the Healthiest Way of Eating*, which is a practical companion to the WHFoods.org website and won 2007 National Best Book Award.

The WHFoods.org website was the first project that George's foundation spearheaded. It was launched in 2001 is now one of the most popular on the Internet when it comes to healthy eating. In fact if you "Google" search "healthiest eating" or "healthiest recipes," the website comes up #1! WHFoods.org has over 12 million visitors per year and was selected as Best of the Best for Healthy Eating in the latest edition of The Web's Greatest Hits by Lynie Arden. And all of this with no advertising as George's foundation has no association with commercial companies. That's why Readers have come to trust the unbiased material George presents because he provides great advice, which is supported by science. Receipts from the sale of our books and DVD go toward continuing further research on and education about the Healthiest Way of Eating.

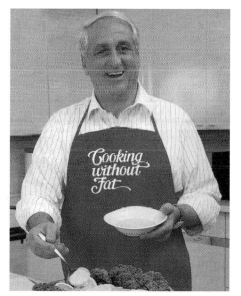

George before he lost 50 pounds

The George Mateljan Foundation

For over ten years, the George Mateljan Foundation been changing the way millions of people make decisions about the way they eat and how they prepare their food

It was established by George Mateljan to discover, develop, and share scientifically proven information about the benefits of healthy eating through the World's Healthiest Foods website (WHFoods.org) and to offer this information to you free of charge. The Foundation is also committed to the publication of books, such as *The World's Healthiest Foods: Essential Guide for the Healthiest Way of Eating*, which are designed to complement the information on the website and provide easy, practical ways to integrate the Healthiest Way of Eating into your lifestyle.

The Independent Perspective

The Foundation is not-for-profit so it can offer an independent perspective that is not influenced by commercial interests or advertising. Its only purpose is to help you discover the many joys and benefits of healthy eating. The Foundation's independent perspective can help provide clear and easy-to-understand knowledge on how people of all ages and backgrounds can achieve vibrant health and energy.

Beliefs

The Foundation believes that true good health is more than just the absence of disease; it is a state where you enjoy all the energy and benefits life has to offer. One of the keys to achieving good health is to use the power of nutrient-rich foods to positively affect how you feel, how much energy you have, and the length and quality of your life. There is clear and definitive scientific evidence that nutrient-rich foods play an important and significant role in reducing the risk of degenerative diseases, and in providing long-term health and longevity.

The Foundation also believes that nutrient-rich foods not only have the power to provide good health, but that they also have the power to provide the pure joy of eating, and the joy of sharing with others. Each individual is unique, so everyone is not fit into the same "food formula." Biochemical individuality is respected and a wide variety of nutrient-rich food options are provided. That way each individual can discover the personalized information, recipes, cooking methods, and menu plans to meet his or her needs.

Our Mission

The George Mateljan Foundation's mission is to offer the latest scientific information about the benefits of the World's Healthiest Foods and the specific nutrients they provide. Equally important, the Foundation offers practical, simple, and affordable ways to enjoy them that fit your individual lifestyle.

Focus: Helping Everyone Learn How to Eat Healthier for Free

The George Mateljan Foundation is focused on using the power of nutrient-rich foods to achieve and maintain good health and the prevention of disease. George has devoted his life to discovering and understanding the benefits of the Healthiest Way of Eating, and because of his passion for helping people, he believes that information on how to achieve vibrant health and energy should be accessible to everyone.

So he has made the Foundation's website, www.WHFoods.org, available free of charge, to anyone interested in learning about the Healthiest Way of Eating.

The profits from the sale of this book go to the George Mateljan Foundation, a not-for-profit organization, which provides funding for research and education to promote the Healthiest Way of Eating and the Healthiest Way of Cooking. The Foundation is dedicated to help make a healthier world.

Other books from George Mateljan and the George Mateljan Foundation.

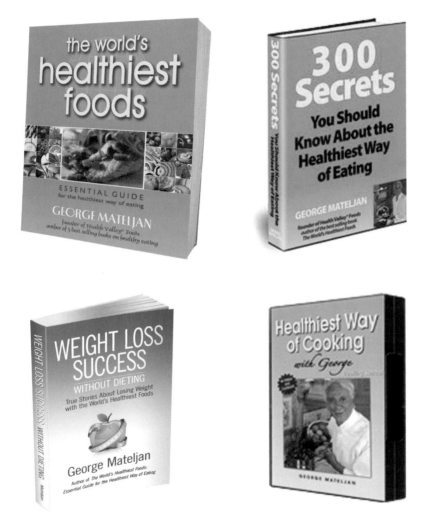

George's Books and DVD are available at www.WHFoods.org